HOMEOPATHY
THE ENERGETIC APPROACH

Michele Iqbal, D.H.M.S., Ph.D.

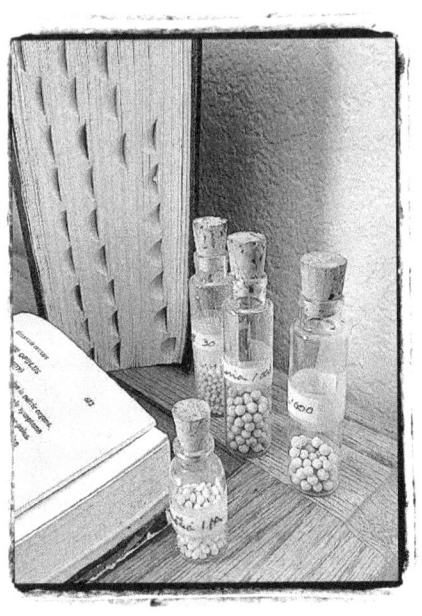

METASTUDIES INSTITUTE
USA

Published in the United States of America

Michele Iqbal,
1735 Spruce Street

Riverside, CA 92507

888-410-1720

First Printing, 2016

Designed by Anita Burns, MetaStudies Institute

Michele Iqbal is not a medical doctor, nor a licensed practitioner, but rather holds a Ph.D. degree in Homeopathy, a D.H.M.S. (Diploma of Homeopathic Medical Sciences) from the National College of Homeopathy in Rawalpindi, Pakistan. The Services Dr. Iqbal offers are complementary and alternative to conventional medical care in the State of California.

" Homeopathy cures a greater percentage of cases than any other method of treatment. Homeopathy is the latest and refined method of treating patients economically and non-violently. "

~Mahatma Ghandi~

Table of Contents

The Energy of Healing is Real.

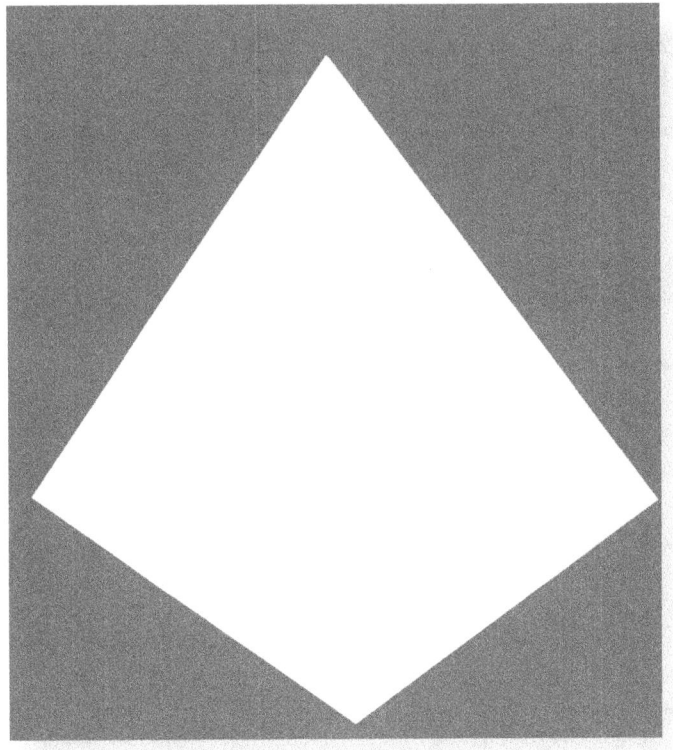

"I am convinced that the sciences are being held back by assumptions that have hardened into dogmas maintained by powerful taboos. These beliefs protect the citadel of established science, but act as barriers against open-minded thinking. (1)"

~Rupert Sheldrake~

Preface

If the human body were as purely material and mechanistic as science has contended over the last four hundred years, wouldn't we understand everything we need to know about human beings by now?

If the sciences are correct in the assumption that the mind is contained in the brain and controlled by chemicals, would behavior be such a mystery? Must there remain a division between the scientific and the non-material nature of humans?

Why must a scientist renounce the roll of unseen energetic structures in nature? Why must a doctor look only at the chemical components of the human body? What is it that has remained a mystery to medicine and hidden from plain view, yet explains that spark of life we all know is there but can't quite identify?

This book explains precisely how energy structures affect the body and how energy medicine can relieve illness and achieve wellness. This is a discipline that I call Thoth-ology, the study of energy medicine's effect on health and wellness.

The word, Thoth, is similar to a word found in Urdu. It describes the idea of a life lived in perfect, splendid contentment—a life not necessarily of wealth and material riches—but rather of wellness, serenity and satisfaction.

Thoth is also the name of a member of the Egyptian pantheon, possibly modeled after Hermes Trismegistus, the fabled founder of Alchemy. By following ancient Alchemical principles—paying attention to the energy fields that animate the material body—and by the use of energy-based medicine, it may actually be possible to achieve that legendary, perfectly splendid existence.

Yet, where did the idea of the perfect life of Thoth originate? Urdu is a language spoken among certain ethnic groups of the Indian Sub-continent. Sir William Jones, a British scholar who studied language and Indian culture in the Eighteenth Century, identified a connection between the ancient Sanskrit language of India and the Greek and Latin languages of classical antiquity. Jones was the first to propose that Sanskrit was the original source of the European languages.

If this is true, and scholars generally accept that it is, then the concept of the perfect life attributed to Hermes/Thoth could have originated in India before it was known to the ancient Greek and Egyptian cultures.

Energy Structures

Knowledge of energy bands that animate the physical body must have originated in India as well. The origins of Sufi Mysticism can be traced to the teachings of ancient Hindu Yogic traditions (1). The description of energy bodies and levels that animate the human body and that control function can be found within the doctrines of ancient Sufism (2). Somewhere in history the knowledge and understanding of these energy structures became separated from hard-core science, yet this knowledge is essential to understanding the human body.

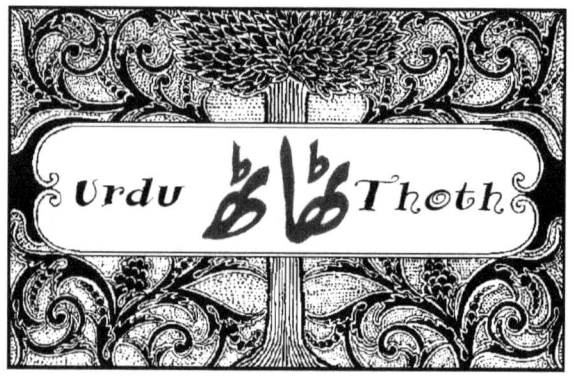

The word, Thoth, is similar to a word found in Urdu. It describes the idea of a life lived in perfect, splendid contentment....

Introduction

I've led an unusual life. My father was a veterinarian and I spent much of my childhood watching surgeries performed on animals. I learned valuable concepts from my dad that taught me to think in unconventional ways.

I married an international student from Pakistan. Since I am an American of Irish descent, that was a pretty radical thing to do—especially in 1972. This was a time when most Americans had had little exposure to nationals from the other side of the globe.

My marriage offered me the opportunity to learn about language and culture from a point of view I could not have otherwise known.

Perhaps the most unusual choice I made for my life was to become a doctor of an alternative form of medicine that has been maligned and ridiculed since the early 20th Century. I fell into this profession because my children were sick in ways that conventional medicine could not cure.

Help came from a man who practiced a method of medicine I knew nothing about. After this physician's methods made such astounding and radical differences in my children, I knew I had to learn more. I felt no one else could care for them as carefully and with as much concern about their health as I would. So I took my first step toward a long and rewarding career in homeopathy that has guided me through amazing but unchartered waters. I completed a Ph.D. Degree in Homeopathic Medical Sciences through the National Council for Homeopathy in Pakistan in 1987. We returned to the States in 1989. I worked for a homeopathic pharmacy in downtown Los Angeles for five years before starting a private practice.

As of this writing, I have been working with homeopathy for over 30 years. Today, I practice in the Riverside area of Southern California. My husband and I have been married for nearly 45 years.

Energy Body Model

For decades I have called myself a Homeopathic Practitioner. However, I practice differently than other homeopaths. I developed a unique system for potency and remedy use based on a model of energy structures present in the human body. It is for this reason that I call what I do Thoth-ology.

Much of the information in Thoth-ology is not a part of classical homeopathy—although the founder of homeopathy hinted at its existence.

The remedies I use are from the homeopathic realm, mainly because the potentizing process is the only process that can produce a true form of energy medicine.

Conventional medicine has been helpful and useful during its four-hundred-year history—and there is much we would not know if scientists had failed to investigate physiology through scientific methods. However, the frustration that millions with chronic conditions feel has led many to wonder if there are as yet unexplored choices in health care.

Unfortunately, many alternative medical modalities are chaotic and unstandardized. The misunderstanding of how a physical body truly functions with subtle energies is the cause of much of the problem.

In the following chapters, I offer a point of view meant to standardize understanding of how our body truly functions as well as the most effective use of energy-based medicine. It is the right time for this information to be known. I feel it is a necessity in the world we live in today.

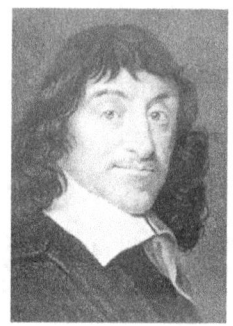

Rene Descartes (1596-1650)

" Rene Descartes (1596-1650) was the principal proponent of the material and mechanistic philosophy of nature and was the first to extend the idea into the realm of life. (1) Before Descartes, scientists followed the views of Greek philosophers—that the soul not only exists, but actually shapes the body (2)." ~Rupert Sheldrake~

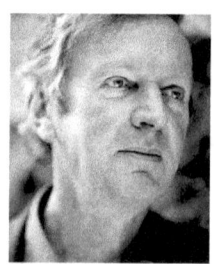

Rupert Sheldrake (1942 -)

Expand Awareness into All Dimensions

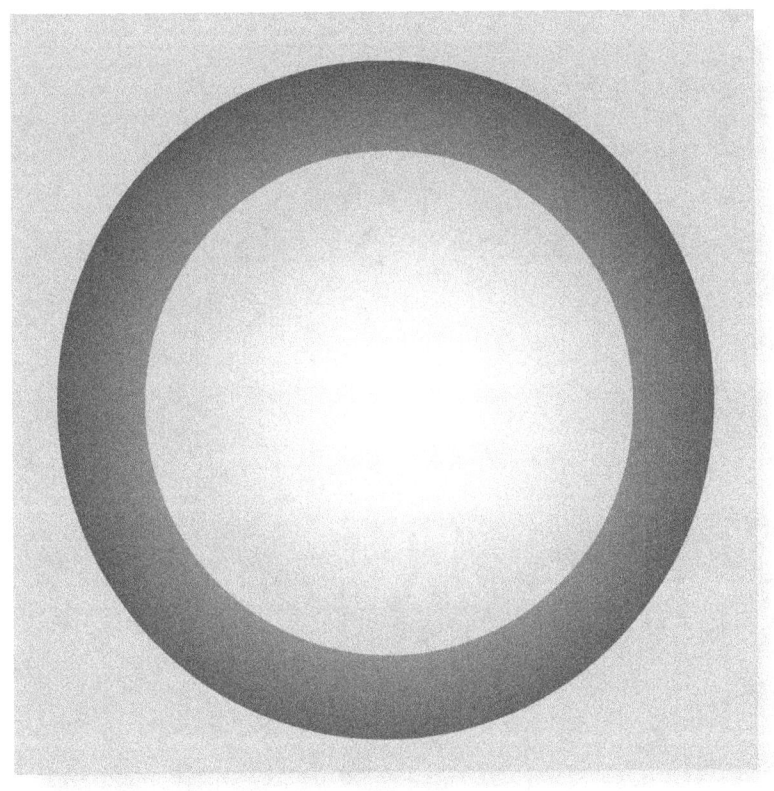

Thoth-ology 101--Basic Principles

Man is not matter. Man is not all soul. Soul and matter go together. Balance has to be maintained.
— Allama Muhammad Iqbal, Philosopher, 1908

Chapter 1

The Materialistic View

Before the great religious wars of 17th Century Europe, science accepted the existence of the soul. The conflict over science versus religion caused the two ideologies to separate.

If this had not occurred, medical science might have remained under the control of the church and unable to move forward and expand. Religious dogma and the crime of heresy stood in the way of scientific progress at one time. However, in the 21st Century it is the scientific dogma of materialism that stands in the way of progress.

Importantly, the Neo-Platonic ideas of the Greeks also influenced Homeopathy founder, Samuel Hahnemann. For part of his life, Hahnemann made his living by translating ancient Greek texts into German. It was during this time that he re-discovered the principles that became the basis of his new medical system

(3). In 1810, he wrote about a dynamic vital force in his book The Organon of Medicine.

Paragraph #9 of *The Organon of Medicine* reads:

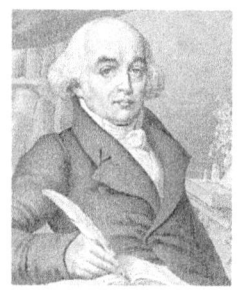

"In the healthy condition of man, the spiritual vital force, the dynamis that animates the material body, rules with unbounded sway, and retains all the parts of the organism in admirable, harmonious, vital operation, as regards both sensations and functions (4)."

Samuel Hahnemann
(1755-1843)

Much of our present day beliefs about science and medicine as material and mechanistic have been the result of historic events that shaped philosophical paradigms and drove experimentation toward the physical and the visible world.

"Atoms are not inert particles of stuff, as in old-style atomism. Rather, as revealed by Twentieth Century physics, they are structures of activity, patterns of energetic vibration within fields (5)."
~Rupert Sheldrake

Cell Energy

Rupert Sheldrake identified the fact that all physical structures are surrounded by a field he calls a "morphic" field, that is in resonance with other fields around other physical structures.

"This hypothesis applies to all self-organizing systems, including atoms, molecules, crystals, cells, plants, animals, animal societies. All draw upon a collective memory and in turn contribute to it (6)." Rupert Sheldrake

Resonance means that these fields are in constant communication. There is an information exchange that impacts form and function of all components of the physical world, right down to the smallest atom. It is this information exchange that Sheldrake calls "Morphic Resonance".

This means that a field of energy surrounds every atom. A field of energy surrounds and interpenetrates every molecule. Likewise, a field of energy surrounds every living cell—and this field is responsible for the cell's proper formation as well as its proper function.

According to Sheldrake, there is an information exchange. "Morphic resonance involves a transfer of form or in-form-ation rather than a transfer of energy" (7).

Every tissue and organ in a living organism is made up of cells. Therefore, an energetic field surrounds that tissue and carries its own resonance, form and function. Ultimately, the entire living organism is surrounded by morphic fields that are in resonance with every tissue, cell and molecule of the body.

These morphic fields are also in resonance with other organisms. Organisms are in resonance with other groups of organisms such as those found in, and among, families, friends and colleagues. Human organisms are also in resonance with other races and other nations of organisms—and even other dimensions where organisms exist.

The Alchemy of Cells

In his groundbreaking book, The Biology of Belief, biologist Bruce Lipton talks about the functions of living cells and how they can be compared to the functions of silicon chips (8). Lipton describes an experiment done in Australia in 1997 in which gold foil was used, along with an electrolyte solution, to stimulate electromagnetic activity in a living cell. Lipton cites this experiment as proof of a cell's comparability to a computer chip. "The second corollary insight is that the programmer lies outside the computer/cell. Biological behavior and gene activity are dynamically linked to information from the environment, which is downloaded into the cell (9)."

What I find interesting in this experiment is that gold is linked to the enhanced function of cells. Silicon chips have layers of gold infused onto the surface that help in the transmission of information across the chip. Gold never rusts or oxidizes and is an electrical conductor when present in the proper concentration. Therefore, it would seem that gold is an important element in the proper function of cells and the programming of cells through our DNA.

This is in line with alchemical principles where gold was used to enhance good health and longevity. However, gold must be converted to a usable form by another metal before it is diluted into an energy state. Otherwise, gold on its own, or in the mono-atomic form, can create problems.

DNA, in the nucleus of a cell, is actually a receiving device that can be compared to the hard drive on a computer that stores programmed information. It can be impacted by information coming from outside the cell, and works best when the nutrients that enhance its function are in the proper concentration.

....gold foil was used, along with an electrolyte solution, to stimulate electromagnetic activity in a living cell.

An engineer who services equipment that makes silicon-processing chips, once told me that there is a limit to how small the chips can be made. If they are made too small, the information gets muddled and the chip doesn't work. However, our computer devices continue to get smaller and smaller because engineers have found a way to stack the chips so more information can be stored in less space. This is similar to the stacking of genetic material on the double helix structure of DNA.

Homeopathy is wholly capable of satisfying the therapeutic demands of this age better than any other system or school of medicine.

--Charles Frederick Menninger, M.D., Funder of the Menninger Clinic.

Chapter 2

The Aura

Today, many branches of metaphysical philosophy refer to the energy that animates the physical body simply as the

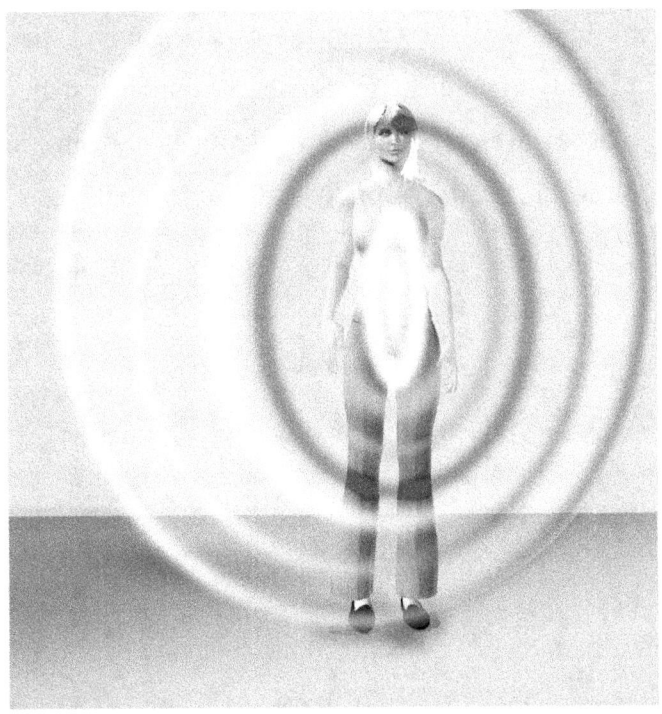

Aura. Scientific evidence of the Aura is hard to come by since photographic techniques often used to prove the existence of Auric fields have become controversial. However, no one who works in energy healing modalities can deny the reality that energy fields exist and are responsible for animating the material body.

The Aura of each individual is unique in frequency and no two people are entirely alike. The Aura reflects the physical, emotional, mental and spiritual aspects of the individual entity that has influence on the physical has often been called the "soul." Science may still argue whether the soul exists, but how would anyone dispute the existence of something spirit-like being present in an individual, whether it be called a soul of something of another name?

In my philosophy, based on life experience and study, the soul is an entity of pure energy. Sometime during gestation, that entity enters a developing fetus. In order to create influence and animation within the developing child, energy bodies form.

Energy Bodies 1-4

The first four energy bodies are present at birth and responsible for our automatic physical functions—such as heartbeat, digestion, elimination and such.

Energy Body 5

The fifth energy body begins to form soon after birth and is the first to cross the skin barrier. It carries information we inherit from our genetic line and the expression of genetic material. That is why inherited characteristics often show up as chronic skin problems.

Energy Bodies 6-10

The sixth through the tenth energy bodies separate us from other animals. All animals have the first four or five energy bodies, depending on the species. Domesticated animals have learned to pattern their energy bodies after us and intertwine their auric fields with ours. This intertwining has become more pronounced over the last few decades to the point where our pets have become family members. A wild animal cannot and will not ever become tame—no matter how they are treated or raised. A wild animal does not have the ability to pattern their energy bodies to mesh with human energy bodies.

Energy Body Development

What follows is a general guideline for the development of energy bodies. Individual experiences, cultural influences and societal norms may influence the age at which these structures form.

- The sixth energy body forms between the second and third year and directs us in becoming independent from our parents and guides us to discover our place in society.

- The seventh energy body normally develops between the fourth and fifth year. This body governs our ability to acquire knowledge.

- The eighth energy body, forming between the sixth and seventh years, is responsible for perceptual comprehension and the development of thought patterns that influence learning such as complex calculation.

- The ninth energy body is in place by our tenth year. This structure helps us to socialize and "read" other people. We become aware of a larger world and how society may affect our life.

- The tenth energy body, in place by our twelfth year, governs the development of independent thought and extra-sensory-perception.

A normal person has all ten energy bodies, but information gathered during the process of development is influenced by the experiences and the training we receive during our lifetime. Some disorders, such as autism, can delay development.

... concretized ideas can be seen in prejudicial thinking, where values and prejudices remain static through many generations.

In addition, each generation learns through the experiences of the previous generation. In other words, information is passed on through energy bodies that individual souls model after the parents, particularly the birth mother. This information sharing may create evolutionary progress.

On the other hand, sharing of information garnered from

birth parents can also create concretized ideas that do not change through many generations.

This also means that the energy-body model I outline here will not remain static. Humans change and progress through knowledge acquired from previous generations—or not.

One example of evolutionary progress can be seen in educational curriculum. At the time I was in high school in the 1960's, calculus was not taught before the 12th grade. Now it is begun in middle school in some districts. My granddaughters are a good example. When I was in the first grade, I barely knew the alphabet and reading was only beginning to be taught with simple three-letter words. My granddaughters could read complex sentences by the time they reached the first grade. I was astonished that this much change had taken place in only two generations.

An example of concretized ideas can be seen in prejudicial thinking, where values and prejudices remain static through many generations.

Dimensions of Consciousness

Are there further unseen structures of resonance connected to our physical body? Is it possible structures that vibrate at a frequency beyond detection are actually responsible for the dynamic functions that define consciousness?

Where the mind resides has been a topic of debate for centuries. Sheldrake suggests that "…the fields of minds are within brains and extend beyond them (4)."

My experience tells me this statement is significant. There is an energy field that influences the function of consciousness, but there is also a chemical component to brain function that is dependent on the physical presence of basic nutrients.

The single-molecule-thick layers of metals that make up the brain of a computer-processing chip must be properly placed for it to function correctly. In the same way, the human brain must be able to absorb certain nutrients efficiently to perform specific functions.

If a computer chip is made incorrectly, the computer cannot "think." If a brain is not functioning correctly, the personality and mind can be flawed—even though these are part of the soul entity. There is an interdependence in a complex system of energy and information exchange.

The proper function of the mind is dependent on the proper formation of energy levels.

The Energy Levels

Positively charged resonant fields of electromagnetic "energy levels" (5) touch on and coordinate with levels of quantum information fields resonant in various dimensions beyond the three known physical dimensions.

1. These energy levels are essential to our ability to function within our environment by touching upon pockets of information residing in higher, non-physical dimensions.

2. These energy levels extend beyond physical

parameters and may be the mode of influence recorded as the conscious observer effect on quantum fields. Scientific experimentation designed to prove the existence of quantum energy has demonstrated that this is true. For more information, look at the work of researcher Dean Radin (6)

Positively Charged

A constant exchange of proteins, hormones and chemical molecules from the membrane of individual cells in our body forms a positively charged field of function around each cell.

The inside of a cell is negatively charged, while the outside is positively charged. This happens by a constant exchange of protein "gears" that pass through the cell membrane (7).

The positively-charged energy fields emanating collectively from each cell form the positively-charged energy fields

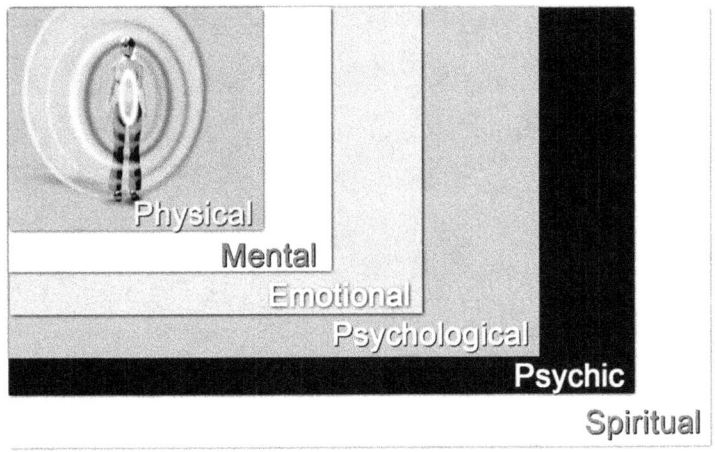

surrounding the macrocosm of the entire organism. This energy field is organized into six levels of function.

All ten energy bodies that animate our physical body lie within the first level—the physical level. Energy bodies are connected to all the levels at all times through Chakra points that emanate from the endocrine glands. This point is hard for modern science to prove, but for centuries Hindu Yogic traditions, Sufi Mystics and Greek Philosophers have described exactly the same concept (9).

> " By tightly regulating the release and distribution of these function-controlling signal molecules, the community of cells would be able to coordinate their functions and act as a single life form (8)."–Bruce Lipton

The First Level-Physical

This level connects the dynamic spirit of the soul to the physical body through the functions of the ten energy bodies that lie within it.

The physical level governs primal fears and survival instincts and develops with the first four energy bodies during the fetal gestation period.

The Second Level-Mental

The second level—the mental—connects us to time and allows recognition of the self in the sequence of time. This level develops along with the 5th and 6th energy bodies beginning soon after birth, but may not be fully functional until much later.

If this level does not function properly, we may have difficulty understanding the sequencing of events—making the individual appear impatient, selfish, or self-centered. Think of the "are we there yet" refrain of small children who do not yet understand the restraints of time and space.

The Third Level-Emotional

This level connects us to the racial and ethnic consciousness of our physical inheritance and governs feelings of patriotism and race membership. This level develops with the 7th and 8th energy bodies that emerge between the ages of three and seven.

If we become stuck at this level, we may find difficulty in seeing the larger picture or interconnectedness of all humanity, leading to prejudicial thinking.

The Fourth Level-Psychological

The fourth level—psychological level—connects to the collective consciousness allowing us to experience an understanding of what is right or wrong in dealing with others. This level would begin to develop with the 9th energy body after age six or seven and should be in place by age ten.

This level governs the development of compassion for others on the planet. Although most people have this level present by the time they reach the age of ten years, it may not be fully functional until after the age of sixty. Many people remain self-centered and think only of what is good for them as an individual until they mature into the fully functional ability of the fourth level.

The Fifth Level-Intuitive

This connects us to the unseen world where inspiration and intuition reside. This is the level that helps us experience a consciousness greater than ourselves.

The Sixth Level-Spiritual

This last level connects us to the highest vibrational frequency of Universal Consciousness. This is the level that takes us from citizen of a particular country and a member of the human race to identifying ourselves as citizens of the universe. This level should be in place by age twelve. However, the full potential of this level remains undeveloped in most of humanity.

All Six Levels

Every living human is supposed to have all six levels, yet each of us may develop the structures within the levels at different stages during our lifetime. Also, not all structures within these levels may become fully developed in everyone.

If, for example, you were a victim of child abuse or raised in an environment void of nurturing adults, you may have problems developing many energy level functions. Certain inherited aspects embedded in DNA patterns may also inhibit the activation process. Individuals displaying symptoms of Autism Spectrum Disorders display deficiencies in energy-level development.

Many of us can be stifled in complete development—or not—depending on the training we receive in childhood. Full activation in all components of the levels can be described as "enlightenment."

Knowledge of these energy bodies and levels can be a guide to using energy-based-medicine.

"...I'd like to point out now that because receptors [on cells] can read energy fields, the notion that only physical molecules can impact cell physiology is outmoded. Biological behavior can be controlled by invisible forces, including thought, as well as it can be controlled by physical molecules, like penicillin, a fact that provides the scientific underpinning for pharmaceutical-free medicine. (1)"

~ Bruce Lipton

I can't manage without homeopathy. In fact, I never go anywhere without homeopathic remedies. I often make use of them.

~ Paul McCartney

Chapter 3

Pharmaceutical, herbal, vitamin, and mineral medicines are material doses of chemicals. Although herbs and vitamins may not be as chemically active as pharmaceutical medicines, they are nevertheless, chemically and physically based substances.

There is only one form of medicine that is truly energy-based and chemical free—and that is potentized homeopathic remedies.

Homeopathic remedies are energy-based and chemical free because of the dilution process. Known as "potentizing," the process converts the molecule from a chemical to a form of quantum energy. Because of this, homeopathy has been maligned and attacked by conventional medical disciplines throughout much of its two-hundred-year history.

There is only one form of medicine that is truly energy-based and chemical free— and that is potentized homeopathic remedies.

If scientists and allopathic medical professionals were correct in their belief that the human body is wholly mechanistic in nature and that only chemical substances can impact it, then diluted substances could not have an impact on our health. However, the mechanistic concept of body function is essentially incorrect. Fortunately, there are signs that the dogmas of science are changing and becoming more inclusive of alternate theories of health and healing.

How Homeopathy Works— Potentizing

Potentizing is the process of rendering natural substances harmless and more effective as remedies. It transforms a substance from the physical molecular state into energy.

The process begins with any natural substance dissolved into a medium and diluted to a ratio of 10% of its original substance to 90% of the dissolving medium.

The medium consists of whichever the remedy substance dissolves into best, such as alcohol, water and alcohol, or lactose.

This first dilution is placed in a small vial then shaken or "succussed" vigorously until completely blended. The result is a 1X potency, also referred as a mother tincture.

Ten percent of the newly succussed and blended mother tincture is placed in a new vial and blended again with a mixture of 10% of the already succussed substance to a 90% ratio of new medium and again succussed vigorously. This is a 2X potency.

Ten percent of this 2X succussed substance is diluted again

with another 90% ratio of medium in a third vial and again successused. The resulting mixture is a 3X potency.

This process of mixing the newest resulting potency to the same ratio of new medium with further succussion is continued to greater and greater dilutions.

At the twenty-fourth vial of blended and succussed mixtures, there are no measurable molecules of the original substance. However, the energy inherent in the original substance molecule has been expanded by the succession and is present in the medium.

Each dilution in the succession process has expanded and enhanced the presence of energy to a level greater than existed in each previous dilution.

 The further a remedy has been diluted and succussed away from the original substance, the more powerful it is for healing.

How is this possible when there is no substance present? There is a morphic field that surrounds each atom, molecule, substance and organism (2). Each molecule has an energy signature—a unique pattern in its morphic field. What expands in the potentizing process is the energy signature in the morphic field of the original substance. This expanded molecular energy field is what impacts the energy field that surrounds a living organism.

More is Not Always Better

The idea that more is better applies only in the physical realm—and only in specific and limited instances. Although a small amount of a vitamin may be useful, excessive amounts of this same vitamin may be fatal because the amount of vital force energy needed to store and convert it to a useful form may deplete the body's vital force reserves.

Our physical body must convert a material substance into energy in order for it to be used as a nutrient. Sometimes the energy necessary for the conversion is more than our body has available. Energy medicine does not over-tax our body because the conversion to the energetic level has already taken place.

A potentized remedy is already reduced to energy, using none of the body's vital force to convert it. The potentized remedy is not only readily available for our body to use, it serves to reinforce and enhance our vital force.

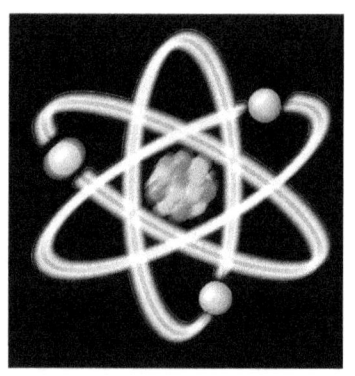

There is a morphic field that surrounds each atom, molecule, substance and organism (2).

More Powerful with Each Dilution

Molecules are composed of atoms in specific arrangements and concentrations. As scientists know, atoms—the basic building blocks of all matter—are actually particles of solidified energy arranged in specific energy fields that have unique energetic signatures. These molecules can combine with other molecules to form various substances known as compounds—each with its unique energetic signature. It is the uniqueness of this energy signature that accounts for the ability of the substance to interact in energy fields and bring about specific changes in those fields.

When energy is enhanced in a molecule or compound by vigorous shaking, the energy field of that molecule or compound is expanded while keeping its unique arrangement and energy signature.

Our physical body must convert a material substance into energy in order for it to be used as a nutrient.

In order for this expansion to take place, a neutral medium, such as alcohol or lactose, which can be absorbed into the molecular energy pattern, must surround the molecule to allow the original molecule's signature to expand without hindrance. This is the basic concept behind the potentizing process.

Energy Expands

When a substance, even an inert one like sand (pure silica sand is ground with lactose until it is soluble in liquid) is placed in a bottle at a dilution of 10% to 90% of the neutral medium—alcohol or lactose—and succussed, the energy signature inherent to the substance is released and expands as it absorbs the medium.

After all the medium has been absorbed by the expanding

energy, further succussion will have no additional effect on the strength of the remedy as it cannot expand further until new medium is added.

This first product is a 1X potency. Each time the material is prepared in this way, it is known as a potentized substance, commonly called a "potency."

Each molecule has an energy signature—a unique pattern in its morphic field.

Through succussion (shaking) the energy expands into the medium, no matter how many molecules there were to begin with.

In the illustration below, the empty circles represent the alcohol medium. The solid (blue) circles represent the molecules of the original remedy substance.

In the second dilution, 10% of the first bottle is placed in a bottle with 90% more alcohol. The mixture is succussed twenty times.

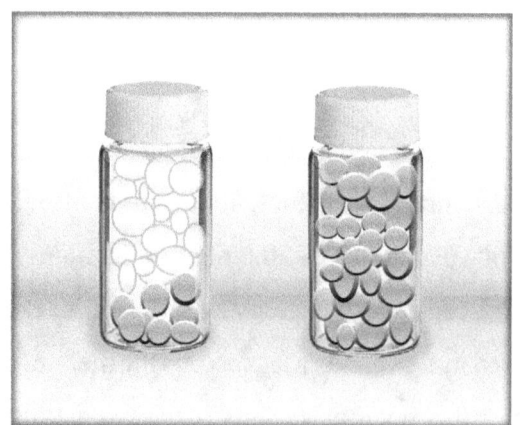

Through succussion (shaking) the energy expands into the medium, no matter how many molecules there were to begin with.

As the new medium is added and absorbed, the energy signature of the original molecule continues to expand until all of the newly added medium has been absorbed.

As this process is repeated in the next bottle, the same thing occurs. The energy signature from the previous bottle expands by absorbing the new medium when succussed. The second product is known as a 2X potency.

This process can be repeated again and again. Each time new medium is added, the energy signature expands even more. As the energy signature expands, it becomes larger and more powerful than it was in any of the previous potencies. Each time the material is potentized, the number before the X is increased by one, indicating the number of times the material has been processed. The X in this case represents the dilution of 10% to 90% on the decimal scale.

It is important to understand that it is not the process of diluting the material, nor is it simply the action of shaking the material that increases its strength. The strength of the potentized material is enhanced by the interaction between these two events.

A substance is placed in a neutral medium that can be absorbed into the original energy signature, thereby, allowing that signature to expand. The process of shaking the material causes this absorption to take place.

Neither of these actions in and of itself, performed alone, has any effect on the strength of the potentized remedy.

The expansion of molecules not only makes the remedy more powerful for healing, but also governs which energy structure that surrounds and controls the physical body the potency will impact most.

Potentization

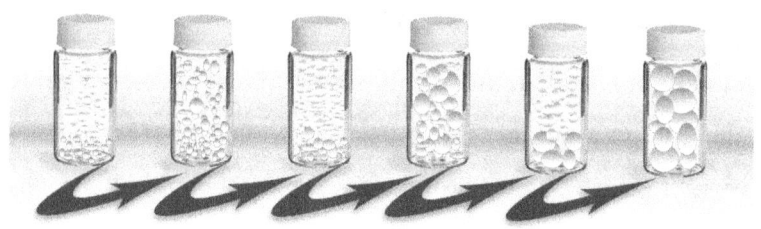

It is important to note that the body can utilize a substance converted to energy when the physical form of the same substance cannot be of use—as is the case with poisons. This occurs because the amount of vital force needed to convert a material substance to an energetic form exceeds our body's vital energy capacity or capability (the poisonous substance exhausts our vital force).

Because a potentized substance is not in its chemical form, it cannot affect us on a chemical level. You cannot be poisoned by a potentized substance even if that substance is chemically poisonous in a material form—as long as the potency is greater than a 6C or 9X potency.

Chemically inert substances or those unavailable for use by our body in their original material form will work in a potentized form. An example is sand. Pure silica, the main component of sand, is the substance that allows a plant to hold up against the wind. If you are low in silica, you will have trouble standing up to the pressures and winds of life's changes.

By taking potentized silica, Silicea in Latin, the problem is corrected. Silica would do nothing if you ingested sand in its physical form.

Caution: Homeopathic Silicea cannot be used by anyone with replacement hardware in the body. Silicea will expel any foreign object.

Potentized Energy Becomes a Remedy

The molecular pattern of a substance becomes an energy pattern that can be used to adjust and modify our energy fields. Based on the rule of "like cures like," a substance that will cause certain symptoms will cure the same symptoms—matching energy for energy, the energy of a potentized remedy to the energy body and level of the illness.

The Difference Between X's and C's

The X and C distinction of homeopathic remedies often confuses users. There are two common forms of classical homeopathic potentized remedies: X potencies and C potencies.

In the potentizing process, if the first bottle is 10% of the substance and 90% of the medium, the potency is an X, indicating the Roman Numeral 10.

If the first bottle contains one percent of the substance and 99% of the medium, the potency is a C, indicating the Roman Numeral 100.

Chemical World vs Energetic World

The key to understanding potency is in realizing the difference between the chemical world and the energy world. Energy has a nature and character distinct from matter.

As a substance is diluted into the energy of a potency, the number of times the medium is changed and the energy expanded further by succussion is what is important.

The potency number: 6, 12, 30, or 200, determines the relative strength of the potentized remedy, not the dilution ratio of the original substance (X or C).

An example of this can be illustrated by comparing two stacks of paper, each with 30 sheets. One stack consisting of paper sheets 8 inches by 11 inches in size—and in the other stack of paper the sheets are 11 inches by 14 inches in size.

If the paper is the same grade, the two stacks will be of equal height regardless of their length and width.

When dealing with the energy of a homeopathically prepared potency, what determines its strength is not how much substance it started with, but how many times it is succussed and allowed to expand into new medium.

A 30th potency of a remedy potentized on an X scale may have started with more chemical substance, but after the 30th potentizing, it is energetically identical in strength to a 30th potency of a remedy potentized on a C scale.

C Potencies   X Potencies

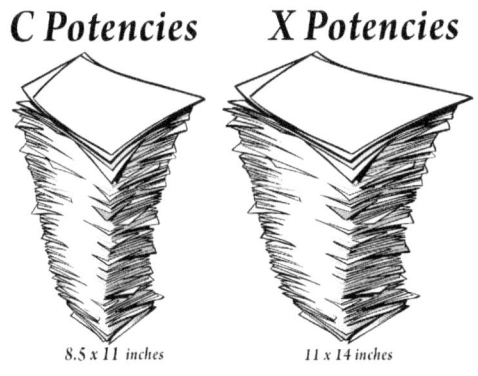

8.5 x 11 inches   11 x 14 inches

The same number of sheets
make each stack the same height

Proving vs Testing

In the homeopathic system, remedies are not tested as pharmaceutical drugs are—they are "proved."

Proving is a process in which a potentized-remedy-substance is given to a person with no particular symptoms. Symptoms that develop during the use of the substance are recorded.

This follows the "like cures like" principle of homeopathy. The symptoms recorded during a proving are used as a guide. The remedy that caused symptoms in a proving is expected to cure a person who is sick with the same symptoms.

Remedies that have been proven in this manner, and are known to be safe and free of side effects, are listed in the Homeopathic Pharmacopoeia of the United States. As long as the remedies used in a combination remedy are listed in the Pharmacopoeia, they are considered safe and will not cause side effects.

These provings have taken place in conjunction with numerous practitioners over a two-hundred-year period.

Side Effects

A homeopathic remedy may aggravate existing symptoms but have no side effects. Aggravations are a sign that healing is taking place. They will always subside when healing is complete or when the remedy is discontinued.

Potency Interaction

How does knowledge of energy bodies and levels impact the use of energy-based-medicine?

There are two aspects of remedies that must be considered:
- The pattern of the molecular-energy signature of the remedy that would be chosen according to the "like cures like" principle of homeopathy.

- The number of times the remedy was potentized— which determines the vibrational level of its action.

Certain principles apply:
- Patterns of malfunction that appear in our energy bodies and subsequently in our physical body as symptoms, will determine the molecular signature that is a match to the chosen remedy (such as Sepia, Calcarea or Arsenicum).

- The time-based origin of a malady will resonate in the appropriate energy level and determine which dilution number (potency) of the remedy is most appropriate. The potency should match the vibrational frequency of the energy level as closely as possible in order to be most effective (6th, 30th, or 200th potency).

- The choice of remedy must match the physical symptoms, while the remedy potency must match the energy level where the illness resides.

Remedy Interaction

As discussed earlier, a Homeopathic remedy is potentized by a series of dilution processes. In the various stages of dilution, the molecule of the original substance is activated and converted to an energy form by the action of succussion.

Each level of potentization in the dilution process increases the vibrational rate of the remedy from the gross in the lower potencies to the very fine in the highest potencies.

The Organon of Medicine describes this process in paragraph #16:

> Our vital force, as a spirit-like dynamis,
> cannot be attacked and infected by injurious
> influences on the healthy organism caused
> by the external inimical forces that disturb
> the harmonious play of life otherwise than
> in a spirit-like (dynamic) way, and in like
> manner all such morbid derangement's

(disease) cannot be removed from it by the physician in any other way than by the spirit-like alternative powers of the serviceable medicines acting upon our spirit-like vital force, ...(3)

The shift in vibrational rate created by increasing the level of potentization must match the vibrational frequency of resonance in corresponding energy body fields and levels in order for the remedy to act most effectively.

6th Potency

The 6th potency vibrates in the realm of matter and gross density. The 6th potency of a well-chosen potentized remedy will work most effectively on the physical body where changes such as injury or functional disorder occur. The 6th potency can be used quite successfully for mineral absorption such as with calcium and iron—or any of the cell salt remedies.

30th Potency

The 30th potency dilution is less dense and vibrates with the energy body and level that develops after birth as our personality and mind begin to form. It is at this level the practitioner will find problems that originate in inheritance, or what is referred to as constitution. The 30th potency is effective in changing constitutionally-based infirmities.

200th Potency

The 200th potency vibrates at a finer rate and resonates with the energy body and level that forms when we are around two years old. This is the time we begin to recognize ourselves as separate from our parents. It is also when we begin to form language.

Also, problems that develop throughout our life from trauma—physical or emotional—can be cleared with the 200th potency.

1000th Potency

The 1000th dilution (1M) vibrates at an even higher frequency and resonates with the energy level that develops after the age of five—Approximately when we have the capacity to learn to read.

Problems at this frequency may appear as learning difficulties or personality traits that impact interpersonal relationships. Personality disorders may be corrected with use of the 1M potency.

10,000th Potency

The 10,000th (10M) potency dilution is the highest form of vibrational energy that will correspond to an actual energy body and level. This is where the highest levels of intellect and personality form throughout our lifetime.

The 10M potencies can be used to improve intellect and information processing—permanently—with only one dose.

Thus homeopathy is a perfectly simple system of medicine, remaining always fixed in its principles as in its practice, which, like the doctrine whereon it is based, if rightly apprehended, will be found to be complete (and serviceable).

— Samuel Hahnemann

March 28th 1833

6th Potency = Works mainly on the physical body

30th Potency = Works on constitutionally-based problems.

200th Potency = Works on life trauma- physical or emotional

1000th Potency = Works on learning difficulties or personality traits that impact interpersonal relationships.

10,000th Potency = Works on improving intellect and information processing- permanently-with one dose.

John D. Rockefeller lived to the ripe old age of 98 and was known to have his homeopath often travel with him. He said that homeopathy is " a progressive and aggressive step in medicine." ~

— John D. Rockefeller

Chapter 4

How does the potentized remedy work in the energy bodies and levels?

Perhaps, it works by making your body aware there is a problem. The energy signature of the molecular makeup of the remedy, matched to the pattern of a problem in the energy body and level will create a phase shift.

Phase Shift

A phase shift can be described as any change in a vibrational wave pattern.

Potentized remedies are chosen according to the symptoms they are known to have caused in healthy individuals (provings). A person that is suffering from similar symptoms brought on by illness will be relieved of those symptoms with the use of the remedy (like cures like).

Diseases occur in a vibrational pattern embedded in our energy bodies and levels. The remedy impulse is a vibrational wave of quantum energy created by the dilution process (potentizing). A phase shift occurs as these two vibrational impulses meet and the illness is overpowered by the strength of the remedy (relief of symptoms).

Remedy Delivery

Since the time of Hahnemann, the traditional way to take potentized remedies has been to place the remedy on or under the tongue. Hahnemann believed that the remedy stimulated nerves present on the tongue (1). Although this has proven to be an effective way to take homeopathy, how it works has never been fully addressed.

The remedy moves into an energy field in a predictable way according to a match between symptoms and the illness.

The theory of nerve-stimulation as a reason for the remedies under the tongue to work is illogical since nerves are stimulated by chemical-based impulses and remedies do not contain a chemical element. Nor does the remedy enter the blood stream as other pharmaceutical-based medicines may when taken under the tongue, since there would have to be substance in the remedy to enter the blood stream.

This delivery system works because there is an energy portal in this active oral region. Imagine a doorway that swings open in the presence of an energetic impulse allowing the activated molecular signature of the remedy to pass into the energy bodies and levels. The delivery system for the remedy would not matter. If the remedy is in a sugar or lactose pellet, or dissolved in water, the portal will open to accept the energy of the remedy. However, if there is only plain water, or plain sugar with no remedy, or food particles present, the door will remain shut.

This is why the rule of nothing in the mouth fifteen minutes before and after taking the remedy has become an important as well as necessary tradition.

After being placed under the tongue, the vibrational impulse of the remedy will begin to move into resonance with the energy body field and level that matches the same vibrational frequency as established by the number of times the remedy has been diluted and succussed.

For example, a remedy of 30th potency will move into and resonate with the 5th energy body and corresponding level.

Your body tries to reestablish equilibrium,creating a phase-shift and a new state of normal that does not include the illness symptoms.

The remedy moves into an energy field in a predictable way according to a match between symptoms and the illness. The wave signal in the remedy will create non-equilibrium in the energy body field by establishing small dynamic oscillations. At the moment the oscillating impulse of the remedy substance finds its match in the disease pattern, a reaction occurs, which appears chaotic in linear time, creating destabilization and non-equilibrium. This is when aggravations may occur.

When a match is established between the disease pattern in the energy field and the remedy's molecular signature, the dynamic impulse of the remedy overpowers and disintegrates all components related to the illness—similar to the way sound waves shatter a wine glass. This shattering allows a new expression to emerge.

After this, the disease is destroyed and you no longer resonate with it. Your body tries to reestablish equilibrium, creating a phase-shift and a new state of normal that does not include the illness symptoms. Wellness becomes the new state of equilibrium.

Samuel Hahnemann, the founder of homeopathy described the same effect two hundred years ago.

Paragraph #27 of *The Organon of Medicine*, Hahnemann states:

> The curative capacity of medicines therefore rests their symptoms being similar to the disease but with power that outweighs it (#22-#26). Each single case of disease is most surely, thoroughly, rapidly, permanently annihilated and lifted only by a medicine that can engender, in the human condition, a totality of symptoms that is the most complete and the most similar to the case of disease but that, at the same time, exceeds the disease in strength (2).

The discussion of the phase-shift described above is an example of the classically chosen homeopathic remedy, selected according to a match of symptoms express by the disease state throughout the body from head to toe (holistic).

However, there are other viable ways a phase-shift may occur depending on the type of illness present in an energy body structure.

Different Types of Phase-Shifts

As a metaphor to describe various ways remedies can function, imagine musical instruments being played by an orchestra to create the movements of a symphony.

In the first example, imagine one instrument out of the entire orchestra being played out of tune or incorrectly. Think of a single organ system, such as eyes or kidneys malfunctioning.

The proper remedy would be one known to have an affinity with the malfunctioning organ, such as Euphrasia for an eye symptom or a Kali remedy for the kidneys.

In this case the phase-shift will occur by the strength of the remedy in a lower 6th potency acting on the lower vibrational density of your body. It does this by recognizing the disease state—either a functional breakdown or a pathogen. The remedy creates an immune response that leads to a return to normal.

If one musician in each section of our imaginary orchestra is playing badly, or the instrument is out of tune, the piece produced by the entire orchestra will be discordant and the music will not have the intended effect.

In the case of chronic disease where an inherited influence has created a symptom in most every part of your body, the remedy must match the whole-body disease symptom complex.

The disease has become normal and a part of every day existence and its morphic resonance creates a phase so familiar it would be invisible and undetected.

A phase-shift occurs as the energetic impulse of the well-chosen symptom complex of the remedy causes your body to recognize the symptoms of the disease state—thereby invoking a response and annihilating all components of the disease, which in turn changes the expression of the original morphic field.

In this case, the remedy is chosen for symptoms that match the entire symptom complex of the disease over the whole body (the entire orchestra) and given in a 30th potency, three times a day for only three days— not repeated. In this way all instruments start playing in tune.

What if one entire section of the orchestra has a problems? Perhaps the violins are on the wrong page of the music sheet.

In this case, an entire body system will have a problem— perhaps a hormonal imbalance or a digestive tract issue. The remedy must match symptoms of the entire malfunctioning system.

For example, Lycopodium in a single 200th potency dose will often annihilate digestive tract pain. Sepia in a single 200th dose can correct a hormonal problem.

Here, the phase shift occurs by creating an exaggeration of the symptom and causing an aggravation that will collapse the energetic pattern of the problem. In effect, the conductor has silenced the violins.

Imagine what could happen if the conductor became angry while conducting. His mood could change the tempo of the music and influence the tone of the piece.

This is an example of using a 1,000th or a 10,000th potency—depending on the remedy—working only on your mental functions. These high potencies vibrate beyond the physical realm at such a high frequency they are not measurable nor detectable by our senses.

The 10M potency of a remedy such as Natrum Mur. can be given to improve mental processing. A 1M dose of Arnica Montana is useful to process and dissipate fear. Usually this remedy is helpful where fear developed after an emotional injury created agoraphobia. In this example, the remedy is non-local, resonates beyond the physical dimension, beyond time and space and does not affect the body in the usual progression of the disease state.

At this vibrational rate, the energetic signature of the remedy is creating an opening to the intuitive and inspirational sources connected to the highest vibrational energy levels and forming a new mental file for understanding of the mental state. A phase shift occurs as the experience manifests as new behavioral patterns. The conductor bypasses his anger to keep to the tempo.

Taking the orchestra example even deeper, think about the universality of drums. Percussion sounds and beats can be heard in most pieces of music played in cultures around the world.

Just as drums are universal, there are universal remedies that will work for most anyone.

These remedies include Arnica Montana for physical injury, Ignatia Amara for emotional injury and grief, and Cantharis for burns. They act in any potency, but when given shortly after the injury has occurred, in an acute dosing style of every 10 minutes for the first two hours—the injury can be prevented from penetrating inward through the outer energy bodies—thereby lessening and even reversing the physical effect of the injury.

The use of these universal remedies as soon as there is a need will create a phase shift that slows the progress of physical impact before it reaches our body.

The damage from an injury does not usually occur right away. A head bump may not show much bruising until the next day. A burn might not develop blisters until hours later, grief may cause sleep problems days later.

This is because our energy bodies have substance and time is needed for the effects of an accident to penetrate through all of our energy fields and cause the full damage that will develop through time.

The use of these universal remedies as soon as there is a need will create a phase shift that slows the progress of physical impact before it reaches our body.

These remedies are also commonly used to promote healing long after the accident has occurred. In this case the remedy produces an impulse that recognizes an injury has created non-equilibrium in your body and a phase shift occurs as your body attempts to reestablish equilibrium.

For remote healing long after the event, a 6th potency of Arnica Montana given three times a day for a period of one month may help if your body is capable of reversing the injured state.

Energy-Based Homeopathy is different from Traditional Homeopathic Theory

In the past, most Homeopathic Practitioners have chosen homeopathic potencies according to their school's tradition.

For example, the British school prefers 6x potencies. Schools of the Indian Subcontinent tend to use 30th potencies often. The French favor the highest potencies.

However, there appears to be no sound theory to accompany these choices—only tradition.

By choosing potency according to the energy body and level model, the probability of success can be greatly enhanced. The reason behind the centuries-old use of the 6-30-200-1M-10M scale of potencies is because each of these potencies hits on an existing energy field and has a place to reside within the structures that animate our physical body.

Other scales may miss the mark and resonate in between the actual structures where health problems originate—creating inconsistent results.

The energy body/level model is one that is workable and effective. I have had great success with it in my practice.

The rules for taking the potentized homeopathic remedies in the energy body model are different than for taking remedies according to other models.

The most important rule is that **a remedy cannot be repeated during its duration time.** If a new energy input is needed, choose a complimentary remedy or a remedy that follows well. One way to know the duration of action of a particular remedy is to check the *R. Gibson Miller chart of Relationship of Remedies with Duration of Action* printed in the back of most *Materia Medica* books printed by BJain Publishers in India.

Most importantly, **never stop a remedy during the three-day-dosing period and start over.** Once the energy impulse of a remedy begins, and more than twenty-four hours has passed between doses, you **cannot** take that same remedy again. It is best to just stop taking it all together and let it work.

If the remedy is repeated during its duration period, the two energy impulses will clash, causing both to dissipate, which will render the remedy ineffective. If you want to repeat a remedy, use a compliment first to offset the energy impulse of the first remedy. It then becomes safe to repeat the desired remedy.

... never stop a remedy
during the three-day-dosing
period and start over.

Chapter 5

Who was Samuel Hahnemann?

The founder of homeopathy, Samuel Hahnemann, was born on April 10th, 1755 at Meissen, in Saxony, Germany. He was the son of a porcelain painter. His childhood was humble, and he attended Meissen High School by becoming a servant in the house of one of the masters. Hahnemann received a classical education and was a top student in the languages of Greek and Latin.

In 1775, at the age of twenty, Hahnemann began his studies of medicine in Leipzig. He made his living by giving instruction in German and French and by translating English books into German. In 1779, he received his M.D. degree.

In 1782, Hahnemann took the post of parish doctor in Dessau and married Johanna Kuchler.

On beginning to practice his profession, Hahnemann wrote that there had previously been no physician at this place, and that the inhabitants had no desire for any such person. He remained there two and half years and commented that the people probably would have done quite well without him (1).

Hahnemann Quits Medicine

In 1784, Hahnemann gave up the practice of medicine entirely, explaining that the rude and barbarous medical methods of the day disturbed his logical and educated mind, which was trained to expect definite results. He disliked giving compounds, the effects of which were unknown. He explained that he could not accept the loose ways and methods of the existing medical schools, hampered by dogmas of doubt and uncertainty. He could no longer accept the risk of doing injury and turned to chemistry and translation as a means of livelihood.

The family moved to Dresden, where Hahnemann made his living by translating texts into German. He also studied chemistry and medical jurisprudence during this time.

In September 1789, he relocated his family to Leipzig where Hahnemann continued his literary work. Because of his translation of medical text, Hahnemann discovered principles that led to radical ideas. It was while translating from English the *Materia Medica* of the Scottish physician, William Cullen, that Hahnemann discovered statements that spoke about a 'nervous energy' as the determinant of the normal state of the body. Hahnemann began his exploration of this new concept by conducting the original experiments on himself.

During Hahnemann's time, China (Peruvian Bark) was a common treatment for Malaria. By taking the cure for an illness not present in the body, Hahnemann was able to observe that the cure would create in a healthy body the same symptoms it would cure in a diseased body.

From this breakthrough, Hahnemann developed the concept of "like cures like" and the equally important concept of "proving." A proving is administering a substance to a healthy individual in order to "prove" which symptoms it would create, and therefore, would cure.

Hahnemann passed the next six years in experimenting with proving the effects of remedies and recording what he found, eventually using his findings on sick people.

In 1796, in *The Journal for Practicing Physicians*, the most important medical journal of that time, he published his essay, *A New Principle for Ascertaining the Curative Powers of Drugs*. In this article, he first explained the principle of "like cures like", declaring that whatever a drug would cause, it would cure.

Between 1799 and 1811, Hahnemann and his family were impoverished, persecuted, and driven from town to town by physicians and apothecaries who accused him of using unfair practices, secret remedies, and quackery.

Hahnemann's first collection of provings was published in Latin in 1805. Five years later the first edition of *Organon of the Medical Arts* appeared. In this, he carefully explained his new medical discoveries and beliefs, mentioning the word Homeopathy for the first time. His new philosophy was a return to the teaching of Hippocrates that emphasized the need to observe the condition of the patient and make inquiries into all aspects of the illness. Due to the concept of "like cures like", it was extremely important to gather all symptoms present in a condition in order that the proper remedy could be determined.

What is Vital Force?

In his book, *Organon of Medicine* published in 1810, Hahnemann explained that there is a vital force, a non-material entity that governs the physical body. According to his concepts, it is not our body that is ill, but rather the vital force that has been disrupted and thrown out of balance. Disease is not what makes us sick, it is a breakdown in our body's energy or vital force that allows disease-causing entities to enter our energy fields and create the symptoms.

We cannot cure illness by treating our body on just a chemical level, we must use a potentized substance on an energy level—treating our energy fields (or vital force) in a non-invasive, non-harmful way that allows health to be restored.

Do No Harm

Hahnemann followed the dictum of Hippocrates: "Above all else, the physician should do no harm." Hahnemann noted that diluted and potentized substances lacked the ability to cause physical harm and were a safe alternative to the healing practices of the day. As he further diluted and succussed his remedies in the potentizing process, Hahnemann discovered that not only did the remedy become less harmful on a physical level, but also became more powerful on a curative level. It was by successive dilutions and experimentation that Hahnemann created the range of curative potencies familiar to today's practitioners.

Chronic Illness-Miasms

The word "miasma" has been used in past centuries to describe unhealthy vapors rising from the earth and causing illness. Before microscopic organisms were discovered, disease was believed to be caused by bad air, fumes from swamps and sewers, magic sent forth in fog to cause disturbance to the population, even by phases of the moon.

During epidemics, cities would shoot off canons to clear the bad air. Residents would flee to the country to avoid the disease fumes. Since fleeing meant less exposure, or cleaning foul water meant less illness, the idea of a miasmatic cause of illness prevailed for centuries. Only with the discovery and acceptance of pathogens did these beliefs wane.

Samuel Hahnemann took the concept of miasma one step further and used the word miasm to describe chronic illnesses that did not seem to yield to his early dilutions. In Hahnemann's theory of chronic disease, miasms are patterns embedded in our constitution that allow illness to manifest in the body.

Constitution

The word "constitution," when used in reference to health, describes weaknesses present at birth. Even if there is no obvious illness present, our constitutional makeup will describe the maladies that will manifest as problems throughout our lifetime.

For example, if you are born with a Calcarea (potentized calcium carbonate) constitution, you will display a problem with absorption of calcium as a nutrient. This will manifest as a poor immune system that allows recurring ear infections in infancy, or recurring tonsillitis. If you have a Calcarea constitution, you will be intelligent but not a go-getter—tending to be quite shy. You may have a problem with bone density—either breaking bones easily early in life, and/or developing osteoporosis later in life. You may be more prone to developing cancer.

Hahnemann named three chronic diseases he believed were responsible for the constitutional weaknesses that allow for the illnesses that plague modern humans. It was his belief that the ancient scourges of venereal disease and leprosy that had passed through millions of people over thousands of years caused chronic disease (2).

I believe Hahnemann described changes that occurred in the expression of DNA coding due to historic consequences in the ancient past. These changes occur in three ways:

1. That which is passed down in the individual's ancestry.

2. That which plagues all of humankind.

3. That which the soul brought with it into this lifetime.

Psora

Hahnemann uses the word "Psora" to describe the first level of chronic illness. He believed Psora to be derived from ancient leprosy that manifests in modern chronic skin ailments such as psoriasis, eczema and chronic itch.

I believe that Psora is something our physical body has inherited from our ancestors' DNA pattern. Psoric changes in DNA that manifest as chronic disease in the present generation were most likely caused by illness, starvation, fear, shame, persecution, enslavement, or torture that was suffered by members of our ancestral past.

The heavy vibrational frequency of emotions such as fear, hate, loathing and extreme pain can change the dynamic systems that control our body and lead to reorganization of the expression of our genetic material.

Syphilis

Hahnemann uses the word "Syphilis" to describe his second level of chronic disease. He believed these were genetic weaknesses originating from the sexual excesses of ancient civilizations that left mankind vulnerable to present day venereal disease—but it is more than that.

I think Hahnemann described chronic illness patterns, that all humankind suffers from, regardless of race, origin, or ancestry, that has led to mental illness and shorter lifespans.

This level of chronic illness could be likened to the Biblical concept of original sin in the sense that all humankind has inherited DNA changes that occurred long ago in our ancestral past.

Sycosis

Hahnemann uses the word "Sycosis" for his third level of chronic illness. The word, sycosis, is derived from the term "metempsychosis" and can refer to the concept of the transmigration of souls. I believe he is referring to the energy patterns that souls have brought with them from other lifetimes.

I believe that a soul's experiences while in a physical body creates a bio-chemical marker that imprints energy structures that stay with us through many lifetimes. This theory is consistent with Sufi concepts of multi-dimensional journeys of the soul through multiple life expressions. These experiences create weaknesses that manifest as personality flaws.

All of these expressions of chronic illness can be impacted by energy medicine—remedies that are processed by homeopathic potentizing techniques.

Healing Takes Place in Many Ways

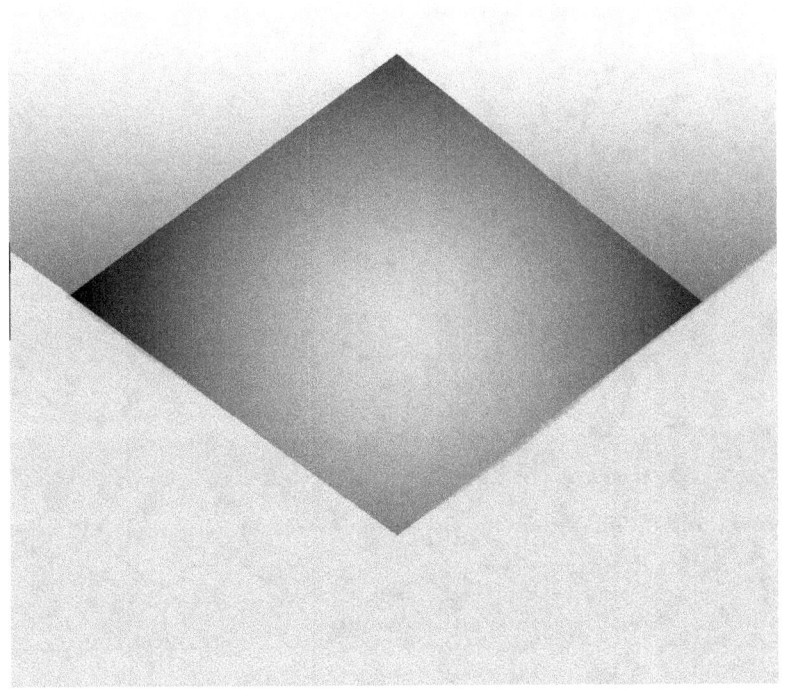

Thoth-ology 102 (Practical Studies)
Therapeutics

"There have been two great revelations in my life: The first was bebop, the second was homeopathy."

~Dizzy Gillespie

Chapter 6
The cases are real. The names are not.

Migraine Headaches

There are three types of Migraine headaches that I have known to be completely relieved by homeopathic remedies.

First: Migraines experienced exclusively by women that recur on a monthly basis and cycle with the menstrual period, or begin at menopause or come on during pregnancy.

Second: Migraines experienced by either men or women that can occur at any age. This headache is often brought on by a reaction to a particular food such as strawberries or chocolate, or due to high levels of stress. The symptoms may include a visual disturbance such as seeing stars, objects blacked out or total blindness for a short time. There is often a stomach upset and vomiting with these symptoms.

Third: Migraines that occur after an accident that included head trauma or whiplash.

My Neighbor's Migraines

When I lived in Islamabad, since Islamabad is the capital of Pakistan, many of my neighbors were originally from other countries. My neighbor Sally was from Australia and we became good friends. During the 1980's, Islamabad was alive with foreign diplomatic families and Sally and I were kept busy with the on-going activities of the ex-patriot community. One of our favorite activities was a once-a-month coffee group that volunteered to roll bandages for the leprosy hospital in Rawalpindi.

On one of those occasions, Sally began to complain that she wasn't seeing very well. I had driven us to the meeting and she explained that she was experiencing the first signs of a migraine headache. Since she knew that her visual disturbance meant that this particular headache would be a bad one, she asked me to take her home.

On the way home, her speech became slurred and she had trouble explaining what was happening. Apparently, she had had a long history with migraine headaches, but I had not known about them until that day. She was concerned because she was pregnant and knew she could not take any medication for the pain. She also explained that the headaches had become frequent during this stage in her pregnancy and she had been suffering quite a lot.

I was in the middle of my homeopathic studies at this time

and I offered to help. She was willing to take a chance on my limited knowledge, knowing that homeopathy would not harm her or her child—and she was desperate for some relief.

I had a small pharmacy of just a few remedies. I remember searching through the Homeopathic *Materia Medica*—the book that lists remedies and their symptoms—to find a match for the headache pain. The remedy I chose to give her didn't work, even though I thought it should have.

She was willing to try again. I don't recall how or why I chose the remedy I did, but I remember just picking one—almost at random—to see if it would work. The remedy was Mag. Phos. 30c, a homeopathic form of magnesium.

She had no idea how casually I had chosen this remedy, but she trusted me and took it. Her headache was gone in record time and she did not have another headache during the remainder of her pregnancy.

This was a fortunate moment for both of us. I have never seen Magnesium Phosphoricum suggested for this type of migraine headache in any of the homeopathic literature. I have never heard of another homeopathic practitioner using it for headaches, but every time a client describes to me this problem with migraine headaches that come on when there are hormonal changes such as during the menstrual cycle or during pregnancy, I have used Mag. Phos. The remedy has worked every single time to stop the headaches and keep them away.

How Mag. Phos. Works

It seems that people who suffer this type of migraine are low in magnesium. The deficiency is subtle and not a general health risk. However, the changes in hormonal levels are enough to cause magnesium deficient muscles to contract and cause the pain. In more recent decades, the use of a dietary supplement of magnesium to treat migraine has become more mainstream. However, the homeopathic form creates permanent change and stops recurrence of these headaches.

Potency

Which potency is used is really a matter of convenience for the headache sufferer. A 30th potency of Mag. Phos. can be taken for a three-day constitutional dosing period to correct the problem—whether there is a migraine at the time or not. If one does come on, a 6X potency can be taken to ease the pain. It is also possible to take a 6X potency three times a day for a month as a therapeutic regime, and then take pellets during a migraine episode if one does occur. In either dosing style, the migraines will continue to diminish until they no longer occur.

It is also a good idea to take a dietary supplement of Magnesium in capsule form just to provide the extra magnesium that the cells will be able to absorb after the Mag. Phos. homeopathic dosing.

It seems that cells deficient in a basic nutrient are deficient because receptor sites on the cell wall no longer recognize the mineral as a good thing to take in. The energy impulse of the homeopathic form teaches the receptor sites to open for the mineral. The homeopathic form provides the energy signature of the nutrient, and a 6X potency would provide a few molecules of the needed mineral, but more may be required to ease the deficiency permanently—hence the wisdom of taking it in capsule form as a dietary supplement.

The European

During the time I was working at a homeopathic pharmacy in Los Angeles, a young man from Europe came into the store looking for help with migraine headaches. He told me he was familiar with homeopathy and had used it in his country.

He was in Hollywood trying his luck at becoming an actor. He had been unsuccessful and the stress was causing him to have more migraines than usual. The visual disturbance he experienced as the episode was coming on was to go completely blind for about a half hour. He was upset because recently this blindness had occurred while he was driving on the freeway.

After the half hour of blindness, he would have nausea, then vomit, and finally the pain would come on. At that time, I had no idea what the remedy to stop this type of severe migraine would be. I knew it would not be Mag. Phos. since his gender was wrong and his migraines seemed to be caused by stress.

I researched my Repertory books to match symptoms to remedies and decided to try Cyclamen. He took Cyclamen 30C, three times a day for three days then came back to see me about ten days later. He described an aggravation during the dosing period in which the blindness came on but only lasted for a few minutes. The nausea was there but he did not vomit. The migraine began to develop, but never fully did.

A few months later he returned to say he had been migraine free. Three years later he returned to the pharmacy to tell me he had never again experienced that type of headache. I was gratified to know that the remedy had worked so well. Cyclamen has worked on others with this type of migraine just as well as it did with the young actor.

Brain Damage Migraines

Often, someone with no history of migraines can begin to suffer after an accident involving a brain injury. In the case of brain injury and head trauma, Arnica Montana would be the first remedy in the treatment regime.

If the head trauma was a past injury that took place years ago, Arnica Montana in a 6th potency, taken three times a day for a period of one month could potentially heal some aspects of the trauma.

For a more recent injury, one that occurred within the last six months, Arnica Montana in a 30th potency for three to five days is appropriate. Arnica Montana in a 30th potency can be taken for up to five days because it is a universal remedy with a short duration period.

For acute dosing where head trauma has just occurred, take the 30th potency every ten minutes for an hour or so to prevent injury from penetrating inward through the energy bodies.

Continue taking the 30th potency for a full three to five days to heal injury quickly.

The second stage of treatment would be to make sure that sufficient amounts of calcium are available for the body to use to heal the brain. This is important because it is calcium the body uses to heal brain injury.

The calcium absorption remedy for brain injury victims is Ammonium Bromatum, taken in a 30th potency, three times a day for three days. Follow this with Lycopodium 30th three times a day for the next three days.

The symptom of an irritable feeling under the fingernails is the sign that the body is robbing calcium from the extremities to try and heal the brain.

The symptom of an irritable feeling under the fingernails is the sign that the body is robbing calcium from the extremities to try and heal the brain. If most people who bite their fingernails were to think back, there may have been an injury or blow to the head—perhaps in childhood—that preceded the desire to bite their fingernails. This symptom of nail biting is often a result of past head trauma, but can be a constitutional calcium deficiency.

Another symptom of the body robbing calcium to heal the brain is the development of heartburn and stomach pain. When calcium is diverted from the digestive tract to heal brain trauma, the digestive system becomes too acidic and heartburn will develop.

The Ammonium Bromatum dosing period should be followed with Calc. Phos. 6X, three times a day for a couple of months, along with a calcium mineral supplement of no more than 500 mg per day. Calcium supplements can be taken in conjunction with Calc. Phos. 6x to assure that the mineral calcium is being absorbed into cells correctly.

Chapter 7

Classical Homeopathy

The original and most often used dosing style in homeopathy is what is commonly called "Classical Homeopathy." The purpose of this system is to find your constitutional remedy according to symptoms displayed over your entire body, including emotions. The goal is to find one single remedy—the panacea— that will solve all of your problems.

The single remedy system of Classical Homeopathy started with Samuel Hahnemann and was practiced by the great American homeopathic doctors of the early 20th Century.

Combination Homeopathy

This is in contrast to the combination remedy approach, where more than one remedy is included in combination formulas.

Practitioners generally agree that combination-remedy-formulas influence problems on a temporary basis, usually only while you are taking the formula, whereas a single remedy taken in the classical style can effect permanent changes and complete relief.

Energy-Body Homeopathy

Since my training was in the Indian-Subcontinent school of thought, I have always relied on the classical single remedy dosing style in 30th potencies.

My energy-body model for choosing potency has proven again and again that a 30th potency, single remedy, taken three times a day for three days only, when no other remedy is taken during the three-day dosing period, works best to bring about permanent relief.

If, for example, you take Arsenicum Album for relief of allergy symptoms, choose a 30th potency—30C or 30X. Either will work.

Dosing

Take a 30th potency constitutional remedy by putting 2 pellets under your tongue, three times a day for a period of three days—and stop. Do not take it for more than three days.

The number of pellets in a dose does not matter. It can be one or four. There is sufficient energy in the original remedy dose no matter how many you use. Take the number of pellets you are most comfortable with.

Most of my clients prefer two pellets. One pellet often feels as if nothing is present, whereas more than two delivers more sugar than is comfortable.

Have nothing in the mouth for 15 minutes before and after taking each dose. Food particles in the mouth may inhibit absorption of the energy on the pellets through the portal under the tongue, and even water can shut down absorption if taken before the energy has absorbed properly.

Aggravations can occur but are usually mild and subside within 24 hours, often within a few minutes. If the allergy symptoms appear most prominently on the skin, the aggravation may seem quite disturbing. This is particularly true if steroid creams have been used on the skin during past eruptions. These creams drive the skin symptom deep into the constitutional makeup and Arsenicum will drive them to the surface again. However disturbing this event may seem, it is a necessary process of healing underlying problems.

REMEMBER:

- Take the remedy for three days only—Do Not Stop before the three days is complete and start over for any reason. If you miss one dose, continue. You can crowd the doses into later parts of the day. If you miss an entire day, you must stop taking the remedy, and you can not start over. This is a serious warning. Missing 24 hours and starting the energetic impulse of the remedy in a second dosing period will destroy its action, permanently.

- If you have to stop because you missed a day, don't worry, it will work, even though it might take longer than if you had stayed with the course.

- Do not worry about the amount of remedy taken, it is an energy impulse, not chemical. The amount of remedy taken makes no difference in effectiveness.

- Putting 1-4 pellets in a bottle of water and sipping from the water several times a day is an alternative to placing the pellets under the tongue. I often suggest this for diabetics or small children.

- DO NOT REPEAT the remedy for any reason. Repeating it will cause the energies to clash and dissipate. If this happens, the remedy will never work for you again.

Allergies

Allergies can be a mild expression of seasonal hay fever, common allergies to foods, or more severe allergies that impact everyday life. If you have an arsenicum album constitution, this remedy, taken in the 30th potency, three times a day for three days only, will relieve allergy symptoms in someone with this constitution.

Arsenicum Album, Latin for white arsenic, is one of the most widely used and powerful homeopathic remedies. It is what is known in the discipline as a "polychrest." A polychrest is a remedy whose provings and clinical use are shown to have widespread uses. Polychrest remedies are often chosen as constitutional remedies.

As discussed earlier, our constitutional makeup is the state of our entire being—from head to toe, physical to mental. I think of a person's constitution as the way they were born into this world—determined by a combination of genetic inheritance, expressions from spirit, and the family's mental state.

The constitutional expression of the remedy Arsenicum Album describes someone who is fastidious, always wants his/her possessions in their proper place and has a problem with anyone using, touching or moving their belongings. This characteristic can have various levels of expression, from mild to a serious organizational obsession.

Arsenicum Constitution

In a mild form, this constitution may express fastidiousness in the form of possessiveness for a particular type of personal possession or space. Perhaps a kitchen must be in order, or an office may have everything in its proper place—and yet other areas of the person's environment are not kept this way. A deeper manifestation of this characteristic would cover all aspects of the individual's personal life including appearance.

I once asked a young man if he cared if his roommate touched or moved his things. His answer was a definite, "he knows not to." He fit all the other symptoms of an Arsenicum constitution.

The Arsenicum constitution would also describe someone who is neat and perfectly groomed at all times. This is the man with a perfectly pressed suit and polished shoes—the woman with a nice, neat hairstyle where not a hair is out of place and a stylishly coordinated outfit. Even in California where people are usually casual and rarely dress up, Arsenicum individuals will have a crease in their jeans, neatly pressed t-shirt, and perfectly clean sneakers.

The Arsenicum constitution loves milk. It is the drink that quenches thirst best for these people. If they have been told to stop drinking it for health reasons, they might cut down how often or how much they drink, but rarely stop altogether.

An Arsenicum person will have some sort of fear issue. Not a paralyzing phobia, but a strong fear, nevertheless. It may be about anything—weather changes, earthquakes, financial failure, or public speaking, etc. It is an ever-present fear, but rarely talked about.

Amy's Story

During a time when my practice was not going well and my husband had been laid off his job, I took a part time job at a fabric and craft store teaching knitting. Knitting and sewing are my favorite hobbies

Amy was a young woman I worked with at this store. Even though she was usually at the guest service counter and never at the fabric-cutting table, she had to wear a jacket everyday because the sizing (a starch-like chemical) on the bolts of cloth caused her skin to break out in red, scabby rashes. She also had frequent bouts of sinus problems and a stuffy nose.

Her only exposure to sizing was through dispersion in the air or by bagging the cut pieces for the customers.

One day as I came into work I noticed that the store was

unusually busy. I stopped at the guest service counter to check on my assigned work area for the day. Amy looked at me with weepy eyes and explained that she was not feeling well and may have to go home even though the store was extra busy and she was needed.

I made a practice of not saying anything about my homeopathic experience because I did not want it to distract me from the job I was hired to do. But as I looked into Amy's red eyes I couldn't help myself.

Often, when I am tempted to share my experience with someone who does not know of my professional expertise, I fear they will not understand my motivation or accept the information as helpful. This is particularly a problem for people who have never heard of homeopathy—which is more common that not. Sharing my knowledge of alternative therapies with others who were not open to these ideas risked people developing negative attitudes toward me. At work, it could have affected my employment status.

Fortunately, Amy was enthusiastic when I told her I knew of a remedy that would help alleviate her allergies. She was open to learning more about it. I asked her if she was a milk drinker— she said yes. I asked her if she liked her things to be in order. She thought about it a moment then nodded.

I took out a pen and wrote Arsenicum Album 30C on a piece of paper. I told her where to buy it and how to take it.

A week later, when I saw her in the store office, she smiled and lifted the sleeve on her jacket. "Look," she said, "my skin is clear."

She had taken the Arsenicum remedy and the redness on her skin had healed. She soon stopped wearing jackets and stopped complaining about a stuffy nose. Essentially, she had stopped being an allergic person.

This remedy has worked every time I have used it for an allergy sufferer—as long as the other constitutional symptoms are there to some degree.

Nut Allergies

I first heard of severe, life-threatening nut allergies in the early 1990s after I had returned from Pakistan. When I was a child, and even when my children were young, I never heard of kids who could die from even being in the same room with a nut.

For many years I wondered how this problem had developed—for I was certain it was a fairly new phenomenon. I don't know if Arsenicum Album would work to relieve this allergy because I have not had the opportunity to treat anyone with the problem, but I believe it would.

I have a theory about how the nut-allergy developed. For almost fifty years arsenic has been put in chicken feed to make chickens grow fat more quickly. This makes the meat plump and juicy.

Over the last fifty years, American consumption of chicken has increased over 250%, mostly because chicken went from a luxury food to an inexpensive one. Chicken has become more available because the FDA-approved-practice of allowing farmers to give arsenic-fortified feed to their poultry has halved the amount of time it takes the average farm-raised-chicken to grow and gain enough weight to go to market.

I began to wonder if the long-term ingestion of the energetic signature of arsenic present in chicken could cause a proving situation. After reading the information on the Alliance for Natural Health (anj-usa.org) about arsenic in chicken feed, I was convinced there is a problem. This would certainly explain the unexpected rise in severe allergies.

Because Arsenicum is the remedy that relieves allergy symptoms, the energetic ingestion of arsenic fed to chickens may be producing allergic reactions consistent with a proving. A proving means that symptoms related to a substance are being produced in persons who had no symptoms prior to ingesting the substance. Long term, over decades, consumption of arsenic in chicken meat seems to be producing extreme allergies.

Don't stop eating chicken just yet. It, along with other meats are an important part of a healthy diet. I have never endorsed a vegetarian lifestyle and find vegetarians have a hard time hanging onto proper calcium levels in muscles and bones— which can lead to muscle injuries that don't heal and bone density problems. Even if you quit eating chicken, the arsenic load would remain in your body.

I do not have experience treating nut allergies, but theoretically, it should work for the allergy sufferer to take Arsenicum Album 30C, three doses a day for three days. Arsenicum Album is such an easy and aggravation-free remedy to take, I'm sure it would not be a problem to try it and see if it works to relieve these extreme life-threatening allergies. There is nothing to lose here.

Knowledge through love or intuition means knowledge through the heart....It comes with a surer step, has a higher and more profound air of authority about it and is born of direct and immediate luminousness.

— Allama Muhammad Iqbal, Philosopher, 1908

Chapter 8

The Calcium Connection

The human body is made up of billions of tiny biological cells. Each one is alive and functions as a separate entity that eats, metabolizes, excretes, reproduces and dies. Each of these individual cells has nutritional requirements that keep them healthy and functioning properly. If the inherited code in a cell's memory is unable to recognize certain nutrients as nutritious and useful, the cell will not take it in. If a large number of cells in the body fail to recognize a nutrient as necessary, the entire body will feel the stress of deficiency. The fluid between the cells may be awash with these nutrients, but the cells have to take it in and use it on a large scale for the body to be relieved of the stress.

The Missing Mineral-Calcium

The complex of symptoms related to calcium deficiency is the one I treat most often with homeopathy. This problem appears in more than 70 percent of my clients.

I believe the reasons for this are many, including immigrants who originate from areas where the mineral content in the soil is different from that in the U.S.—especially the British Isles. Florescent lighting, demineralized and purified water, carbonated beverages, and agricultural pesticides may also be causative factors.

When I lived in Pakistan, I did not see anywhere near the same number of people with calcium deficiency problems. In that country, the population has been homogeneous and indigenous for nearly three thousand years and have traditionally had far less exposure to industry-driven environmental issues than the U.S. When I lived in Pakistan, carbonated soft drinks were a luxury and bottled water was unheard of.

This complex of symptoms is marked by a history of recurring infections, beginning with ear infections in childhood. If it is not ear infections, it is tonsillitis, or bronchitis. Sometimes symptoms include kidney, bladder, upper respiratory, or sinus infections. Whatever the site of infection, it will have been recurring throughout your lifetime and chronic inflammation will develop in areas where infection has occurred.

Calcium is a nutrient so important to our body that it controls our response to infection. When you are calcium deficient, infection is a life-long problem and can be deadly without antibiotic treatment.

You might say, "But I'm never sick." On closer examination, however, you will probably discover that you have a history of minor, yet definite, recurring infections. These may not have been severe enough to put you in bed or a hospital, but if they were never completely relieved or became chronic, it will stay with you and worsen your health over time.

Whatever your infection, or how severe or minor it may be, there is always a history of infection when calcium absorption into cells is low.

Another problem you would find is that broken bones and injuries heal slowly. Maybe you would be prone to injury when playing sports, and have a tendency toward forming excess scar tissue.

Calcium is necessary in order to heal injury—not just broken bones, but brain trauma and deep tissue wounds as well. And, calcium holds up the body by strengthening the skeletal structures.

I have seen the results of skeletal calcium loss in sufferers of rickets and osteoporosis. Rickets used to be a disease of the malnourished. Now it is returning in places where nutrition is not in question.

One more piece of evidence that the problem with mineral absorption is now a major health issue—at the time of this writing, children are suffering broken bones at a rate never seen before.

Depression

If you are calcium deficient, you will have a history of depression or feelings of worthlessness due to low energy levels and a sense of hopelessness. Perhaps you have a self-esteem issue or lack self-confidence. Many times calcium deficiency shows up as Seasonal Affective Disorder (SAD). If you find that you are depressed in the winter when there is less sunshine, you will be deficient in vitamin D or unable to produce it or store it in the body.

I have seen people who were depressed from October when, in the United States, the daylight savings time changes to standard time until March when the time changes back. I may see more people with this condition in Southern California than I would in other parts of the country since so many of the sufferers have moved to Southern California for the sunny climate.

Sugar Cravings

If you crave sweets and sugary foods, or stimulants such as coffee, or diet pills, your metabolism is probably on the lower end of normal. Sugar and coffee give a temporary lift to a low metabolism.

Poor Muscle Tone

If you have flabby, toneless muscles that aren't helped by exercise, your poor muscle tone is due to poor calcium absorption. Parents and teachers may have verbally abused you as a child for not trying harder, but attempts to be active yield little or no results.

With this type of poor muscle tone, activities requiring strength are completely undo-able. As a child and even into adulthood, you will have preferred a sedentary life. Movement can be painful, tiresome and worthless. Your skin will be easily prone to pain—even from minor touch. You might even avoid physical contact with other people or not be able to wear tight-fitting clothing.

You are more likely to be the kind of person who would be easily fatigued when attempting active sports, or be unable to perform certain sports due to poor muscle tone. On the other hand, you probably can continue low-key levels of activity far longer than others since your lack of muscle tone limits the build up of lactic acid and other fatigue related chemicals.

Stomach Acid Imbalance

Other symptoms of poor calcium absorption could be a life-long problem with improper stomach acidity. With this, you will be prone to heartburn and may develop stomach ulcers or acid reflux disease late in life. You might be constantly hungry. High stomach acidity creates a situation where food digests faster than someone with a different biochemistry. There is no natural control over eating because your stomach is always empty and burning for more food. You probably rarely if ever feel sated when you have had enough to eat and your stomach is full. You might only stop eating when your belt is tight and your stomach is completely stuffed. You will also most likely have a life-long problem with constipation.

Not all the people I see with this complex of symptoms are terribly overweight, but many are. Some are only slightly overweight and have learned to bypass many of the symptoms enough to control weight to some extent, particularly in their teen years and early twenties. However, obesity can be a problem and become more so as they get older.

The weight issue begins with a low metabolism because a calcium deficient person usually has a low thyroid function. Possibly, calcium deficient cells cry out for the nutrient they are not able to get, even where there is over saturation of calories— causing overeating in an attempt to be nourished. The signal for a full stomach is missing and *....a calcium deficient person usually has a low thyroid function.* the brain never tells you to stop eating because your cells keep trying to get what is missing—or—the message to the brain is not being transmitted. Also, your stomach always feels empty and ready for more.

However a calcium-deficient-induced weight problem may have started, it could have been made far worse with stimulants and diet drinks in attempts to lose weight. Stimulants and non-calorie drinks corrupt body cell receptor sites and insulin signaling pathways—causing weight gain. Often, what started out as "a little weight problem" becomes a huge, morbid obesity problem by the use of such products.

Many people are born with this complex of calcium deficient symptoms. If you are one of these, and your parents do not have the same symptoms, most likely a grandparent did. If they did not show the signs of it from childhood, it could have been acquired from an accident where many bones were broken, or from severe head injury. This is because your body's extreme need for calcium to heal head injury or broken bones--or even minor surgery in some cases, puts the rest of the body in calcium deficiency.

A major problem facing the American people today is calcium deficiency. It is one of the reasons kids would rather spend recess eating than playing. The calcium deficiency that our parents displayed slightly is passed on to the next generation of children where it appears in a more severe form. Each generation displaying symptoms of calcium deficiency is more severely affected than the previous generation.

The body can be awash with calcium in the blood stream or in the fluid around tissue due to supplementation, but if the calcium is not passing into the individual cells of the tissues, all the symptoms I describe here will be present.

Medical science can only measure the calcium in the blood or other fluids, not in the tissue. The cells reject the calcium molecule because it is large and looks to be a foreign object to cells where absorption was interrupted due to ongoing stress that has shut down receptor sites, or the deficiency of an accompanying mineral such as iodine. This is where the low normal thyroid function comes into play.

American soils are notoriously deficient in iodine, that's why it is put in the salt. However, iodine in salt does not seem to be solving all the problems associated with the need to absorb iodine correctly. Incomplete iodine absorption may cause a calcium problem, but the iodine doesn't absorb correctly until the calcium is returned to cells.

Many people believe that taking the gross material form of calcium is all that is needed to prevent the problems associated with deficiencies. Often people will tell me, "I take calcium, a 1000 mg a day, I can't be calcium deficient." This statement reflects the confusion between what is taken into the body and what can be used by the body. Gross form calcium, no matter how much is present in the body, may not be used properly until it is converted into its energetic form.

The actual situation in most cases is that calcium in its whole molecular form is so large the cells of the body perceive it as a foreign object. This inability of the cells to recognize calcium as a nutrient occurs for many people in the U.S. because we are the descendants of immigrants to this country.

Those of us whose ancestors emigrated from the British Isles, the Northern European areas of Belgium and The Netherlands, the fish-eating coastal cultures of Europe, Mexico, and Polynesia are descendants from biological bodies that were accustomed to large amounts of iodine in the food source.

The difference in the iodine levels in the food interrupts the production of thyroid hormones that interrupts the hormones of the parathyroid gland, which in turn interrupts the conversion of calcium to an energy form and absorption into cells. Once this pathway has been interrupted, it does not bounce back to normal easily and usually requires help.

The descendants of residents that originated from the British

Isles, particularly Ireland, seem to be prone to this problem because their ancestors used sea kelp to fertilize the agricultural fields. The switch to modern fertilizers or the import of food from other countries will produce the same iodine deficiency in modern day residents of these areas as it does for residents in the U.S.

Our cells will not allow this calcium molecule to pass through receptor sites on the outer cell membrane, or the body lacks the sufficient vital force memory of how to convert the calcium molecule into energy. In most cases, the calcium you take from supplements just sits in the intercellular fluids and starts to deposit in nodules. These nodules become bone spurs that develop in storage places such as the heels and around joints.

I find that women who overuse calcium supplements are prone to uterine fibroid tumors.

I find that women who overuse calcium supplements are prone to uterine fibroid tumors. In men and women, calcium supplementation can contribute to the arthritic overgrowth of calcium in the joints. Calcium nodules can also deposit in muscles layers causing fibro-myalgia pain.

If you have calcium deposits where you shouldn't, a doctor is very likely to take you off all forms of the mineral, which doesn't solve the deficiency or correct the problem of calcium deposits.

In most cases, the deficiency caused by iodine interruption

does not register as a calcium deficiency on any medical test.

Currently, there is no way to test the calcium level inside cells of tissue. This is the reason why deep-tissue calcium deficiency goes undetected by conventional medicine.

Opening Receptor Sites

By using homeopathically prepared calcium remedies, these symptoms change and the problems disappear. Only a homeopathically prepared dose of calcium, Calcarea Carb. or Calcarea Phos., can open the door of your cell's receptor sites and allow calcium to get in—as well as teach your body how to get rid of the excess, bringing balance.

Only a homeopathically prepared dose of calcium can begin the conversion of the material form of calcium to energy-based calcium necessary to solidify the energy bodies and defense-system-structures.

Calcium is what your body uses to fight infection and kill bacteria through the immune system. Homeopathic Calcarea remedy can stop the infections. This includes ear infections in babies and all other recurring infections.

Over the years, I have often seen children with frequent ear infections, tonsillitis, or some other frequently occurring infection as a result of calcium deficiency. When presented with these symptoms the first thing I think of is homeopathic calcium. With a regime of Calcium based remedies, Calcarea Carb. 30, followed by a couple of months on Calcarea Phos. 6, these children are able to completely get rid of these recurring infections.

Calcarea remedies stop heartburn and stomach symptoms by stabilizing calcium in the digestive tract and balancing the level of acidity. Many times heartburn and high stomach acidity will have started from a head trauma. This happens because your body pulls calcium from the digestive tract in an attempt to heal head trauma, leaving stomach acids more acidic than normal. A head trauma patient who has seizures due to damaged brain tissue stops having seizures and begins to heal by taking homeopathic calcium.

Calcarea remedies impact metabolism. I have seen children who didn't want to do anything but watch TV, want to go out to play after beginning a regime of homeopathic Calcarea remedies.

With calcium absorption, muscle tone improves. Incorrect calcium absorption causes nerve endings to fire off incorrectly...

A child without calcium absorption problems won't stay inside or remain inactive. In addition to becoming more physically active, these children begin to be more interested in school and show a rise in self-confidence.

Adult and young adult clients report the same increase in interest in job or school activity. They willingly increase their physical activity and depression often disappears as does the desire to be in the sun year-round.

With calcium absorption, muscle tone improves. Incorrect calcium absorption causes nerve endings to fire off incorrectly creating a lack of muscle tone—including the muscle structure of blood vessels. Lack of calcium causes an integrity problem in the circulatory systems of the body. Calcium absorption created by remedies such as Calcarea Fluorica in a 6x potency can increase the integrity of the muscle structure in blood vessels throughout the body.

Muscle Tone

Using homeopathically prepared calcium helps body cells absorb calcium molecules correctly. Muscles develop tone and blood vessels improve integrity.

This process can take a bit of time. When it happened to me, I felt a ring of tone begin at the base of my legs and move up through the muscles as if the ring were being pulled upward. My muscles became firm, but it took about a year.

Many people report a loss of inches during this process without a loss of weight. This is because the muscles and bones are becoming denser by converting fat to muscle and bone tissue. You may become slimmer even though it may not be apparent on the scales.

By balancing calcium, you are less susceptible to injury and heal more quickly. It becomes more comfortable to move around and exercise becomes more effective.

If you are athletic and have always had good muscle tone, you would never have experienced any of the symptoms of this complex.

A homeopathic regime of Calcarea and other calcium absorption remedies will change the symptoms, but the situation does not change permanently without dietary supplementation of elemental calcium—nor does calcium absorb correctly without the use of the homeopathic forms. The homeopathic diluted form of calcium teaches your cells to again absorb calcium molecules. Your cells relearn to absorb calcium and your symptoms disappear. Only a combination of the homeopathic form in conjunction with the dietary calcium will work. However, only a small amount of the dietary supplement of calcium is needed.

Change Takes Time

The kind of change homeopathy can offer is permanent. This takes time and patience. You will need to follow a regime that takes a few remedies and a certain amount of time. Many changes will be apparent immediately, but this does not mean it is time to stop taking the remedy.

The full extent of the remedy will not be apparent right away, but how long the remedy will take is different for each individual. The good news is that regardless of diet, lifestyle and environmental factors, changes in well-being and improvement in overall health do happen.

Calcarea is Latin for Calcium

All homeopathic remedies are written in Latin to distinguish them from pharmaceuticals and herbals. Calcarea remedies are derived from calcium and converted to energy by dilution and succussion. Calcarea remedies address all the symptoms of a calcium deficiency and relieve problems associated with it. The complete list of Calcarea related symptoms can be found in the *Handbook of Homeopathic Materia Medica with Repertory* by William Boericke, BJain Publishers, India.

The Calcium Absorption Regime
can be found in Chapter 10

Chapter 9
Clinical Results

Fibromyalgia

Fibromyalgia is a painful condition that has become all too common in the modern world. Often considered a psychosomatic illness, fibromyalgia is characterized by sore achy muscles that hurt from the slightest movement.

Psychosomatic is defined as an illness where emotional factors bring on physical symptoms. A peptic ulcer could be considered psychosomatic. When the emotional factor is removed, the ulcer usually gets better. Fibromyalgia pain usually does not get better with removal of the emotional factor. It is far too common in our busy world because it is the result of high levels of stress, emotional upset or stress over an extended period of time—and too much calcium supplementation.

When you experience an emotional upset, a stressful

situation, or become angry, you will tense your muscles in response. This causes a slight injury in the deep muscle tissue. Your body sends calcium to heal the injury, but if your body cells are not absorbing calcium correctly, once the calcium crystals are placed in the muscle for the healing process, they are not reabsorbed again. These seemingly helpful crystals remain in your muscle tissue and continue to irritate with the slightest movement. Over time, the pain becomes unbearable.

I have successfully treated this condition many times. Calcium absorption remedies take care of the problem by encouraging the cells of the muscle tissue to absorb the calcium crystals. The calcium crystals are absorbed and the pain goes away.

Susan, a sixty-ish woman I had known for a while, had been widowed at an early age and was struggling with financial issues. Whenever an alternative practitioner, such as an acupuncturist or a chiropractor, gave a presentation in the group, Susan would ask if there was a treatment for fibromyalgia. The answers were usually vague or described as long-term treatments. Because of her finances, Susan never attempted any of the suggested treatments.

One day, I told her that I knew a homeopathic treatment for her pain. She hesitated and told me she had tried homeopathy one time but that the prohibitions about not eating mint, chocolate, or anything with caffeine, and no coffee—ever—were too much for her to handle so she could not use potentized remedies.

I explained that those prohibitions had come down in the

homeopathic profession through long standing traditions and that if everything on the list truly worked as antidote, no one would have benefited from the use of remedies over the years.

I told her that I employ a different model for using potencies that doesn't prohibit any foods, not even mint in toothpaste, or coffee, and that I have had a lot of success with relieving fibromyalgia pain. Susan came to my next low-cost clinic and began to find relief with her first regime of calcium absorption remedies.

Depression

I once treated a man who described severe seasonal affective disorder (SAD). Bob would become depressed in the fall when the daylight savings time changed to standard and the days grew shorter until the spring when of daylight-savings time returned. Even in Southern California where there is little rain most years, where cloudy weather does not last long, Bob felt severe depression just from the difference in the length of day through the winter months.

I explained that there are several calcium absorption remedies to choose from, but in the case where seasonal depression is present, the remedy is Ammonium Carbonicum instead of Calcarea Carb.

Ammonium Carbonicum targets the skin and the inability to properly produce or hold onto vitamin D, which may be due to the lack of calcium in skin tissue. The Ammonium Carb. constitution also describes a person who is often cold, doesn't want to get into water because it is so chilling, or doesn't want to change clothes because becoming undressed causes a chill.

These symptoms occur in varying degrees, and most people with SAD will endure a chill in order to bathe and change into fresh clothes. Other habits, however, may be more telling, such as an unwillingness to swim or wearing a favorite set of clothes most of the time.

Someone with this disorder, who is a candidate for Ammonium Carb. will have extremely sensitive skin. They might not like to wear a watch or a ring, or perhaps they stay away from crowds to avoid being touched.

A three-day course of Ammonium Carb. 30, followed by a three-day course of Lycopodium 30, completely cleared away Bob's SAD .

I always follow a calcium absorption remedy with Lycopodium because it sets-in the calcium absorption lesson so that cells continue to reliably absorb calcium molecules.

Childhood Ear Infections

The problem of recurring childhood ear infections is easily solved with any calcium absorption remedy in any potency. Calc. Phos 6X works well. The pellets made by the Hyland's company are soft and easy to use with even the tiniest baby. Just put one pellet on the child's tongue a couple times a day for a few weeks and the recurring infections will cease.

If a new infection does occur, repeat the dosing period. The infections will stop. As an added bonus, this 6x remedy will help strengthen the child's permanent teeth as they form under the gum.

Bone Density Problems

Ellen, a woman in her 80s, came to me because her doctor had discovered she had severe osteoporosis. I put her on my calcium absorption regime, and after two years her bone density had improved 13%.

"The introduction of homeopathy forced the old school doctor to stir around and learn something of a rational nature about his business. You may honestly feel grateful that homeopathy survived the attempts of the allopaths to destroy it."

Harper's Bazaar , 1890

—Mark Twain

Chapter 10
The Program

Everyone loses calcium through some source: aging, harmful environmental exposure, stress, physical trauma, unhealthy diet, or because we came into the world calcium deficient due to our immigrant heritage.

Restoring calcium improves your ability to heal injury, maintain immunity, stop recurring infections, and possibly stabilize weight. Everyone can benefit from a healthy calcium level.

Using homeopathy changes your body functions—permanently, without pain or mental effort. Yes, this takes some time but it's generally pretty effortless and the changes are often dramatic.

If you start the Program now, in a year you will be an entirely different person, dramatically better and healthier. If you never start because it seems too complicated, too expensive, too long, or too slow, where will you be in a year? You will still be calcium deficient.

What have you got to lose? Hidden weaknesses, emotional baggage and nutrient deficiency.

What do you have to gain? Your good health—plus a whole new sense of well-being and mental clarity.

The First Stage

Schedule for Making Permanent Changes:

This remedy schedule may only need to be done once, or tuned-up after a few years if you experience injury, surgery, or extreme emotional shock—or if you use stimulants to lose weight or consume energy drinks that contain ginseng or other herbal energy enhancers. The habitual use of stimulants will shut down receptor sites on cells closing off your ability to absorb calcium and other nutrients, resulting in weight gain and calcium absorption deficiency.

If a new problem with calcium absorption arises, you can repeat the remedies if you experience symptoms such as recurring infection, sweet or salt craving, or high stomach acidity.

All of these remedies are taken alone for a period of only three days. Whether it is 30x or 30c does not matter—even if you follow a 30c with a 30x remedy. What matters is that it was diluted 30 times, not which scale was used in the process.

In order to use a 30th potency, purchase a 30th potency. NEVER attempt to add up potency numbers by taking more than the recommended dosage at a time—that doesn't work. Two times the dosage of a 6X does not equal a 12X. It just means you have taken a lot of the 6X—which remains a 6X.

Taking two different potencies to equal a 30th potency does not work. I emphasize this because clients have told me that they have been advised by unknowing health food or vitamin store employees that buying and taking a 6th and a 15th at the same time will add up to a higher potency. IT DOES NOT. Taking two different potencies at the same time creates drainage, not the effect you want. **Only a 30th potency is a 30th potency.**

There is no difference in taking one pellet or the whole bottle at one time. The amount of remedy does not change the potency of the remedy in any way.

Due to the homeopathic rules of compatibility and the relationships between remedies, many homeopathic remedies must be taken in a specific order. If not, their effectiveness can be severely compromised.

Many remedies act over a long time—some for up to 60 or even 90 days after they are taken. That is why they are taken in a complementary order.

Remedies must be allowed to continue to work in conjunction with each other in a beneficial way. You will not be harmed if you take them out of order, but one remedy can ruin the effectiveness of another and increase the possibility for aggravations.

Remedies absorb through an energy portal under the tongue—not into the blood stream as previously thought. In order for this absorption to take place, there must be no food particles in the mouth.

- Before taking a remedy, be sure there has been nothing in your mouth, including water, for 15 minutes before putting any remedy under your tongue.

- Wait another 15 minutes after taking the remedy before allowing anything else in your mouth.

A dose is usually 2 pellets. The alcohol used to potentize a remedy is put on sugar pellets for easy use. A dose of 2 pellets makes a good coating under your tongue. However, if you are diabetic, or want to conserve the pellets for some reason, put one or two pellet in a bottle of water—any size—and take sips as a dose.

Remember, this is an energy impulse to energy bodies and not a material, chemical-based medicine. One pellet is a dose, as well as the whole bottle is a dose if taken at one time.

Energy rules apply here, not the rules of substance building in the blood stream. If a child eats the remedies, don't worry—even if they consume an entire bottle. Remember, to a body that does not need the remedy, the preparation is only sugar or lactose.

If the instruction is to "Wait a few days after taking a remedy," this means that you shouldn't take another homeopathic remedy for three to four days, or longer, after finishing the three-day course of a 30th potency remedy. The time does not have to be specific or exact, use your own judgment as to how you feel or want to proceed. Just keep in mind that allowing more time for a remedy to work alone before another remedy is introduced is always a good thing with homeopathy. For example, if you have to wait for a mail delivery before you can begin your next remedy, no harm is done.

You may continue to take any prescribed pharmaceutical or herbal medicine while taking a homeopathic remedy. Since pharmaceuticals and herbs are chemical-based medicine and homeopathy is energy-based, the two forces never meet.

In spite of what you may have heard, it is all right to continue a homeopathic remedy alongside your regular medication. Ask your doctor about this regime if you are on multiple medications or suffer a serious illness.

Understand that if you do choose to follow this program of homeopathic remedies, it is of your own accord. I am imparting knowledge that I have gained over many years of experience in the hope that others benefit from what I have learned, but I am not a medical doctor and I am not forcing anyone to do anything against their better judgment. I cannot be held responsible for any perceived harm that may result from the use of these remedies, nor for the lack of results, since many factors undetectable and not related to homeopathy may be at cause.

Homeopathic remedies are energy-based and do not impact directly on the physical body. A homeopathic remedy cannot cause or aggravate a situation that is not already present. I am not responsible for the misunderstanding of these concepts if the previous chapters have not been read or understood by the individual.

Do not choose homeopathy over the advice of your regular physician. Homeopathy does not replace the treatment your doctor may have already recommended, but homeopathy may be used as a complement to regular treatment if your doctor so agrees.

Sodium and Calcium Absorption:

Remember, each remedy in this program is to be taken alone, for a period of **three days only.** After completion of the three days, go to the next remedy. That means, Natrum Mur 30th potency is taken alone, three times a day for a period of three days. At the completion of this three-day-period, go on to Calcarea Carb.

Be sure to take each dose only if you have had nothing to eat or drink for 15 minutes before. Wait 15 minutes after taking each dose before eating or drinking anything.

Regime for Sodium and Calcium Absorption:

1. Natrum Mur 30th potency – 2 pellets, three times a day for three days. Wait two-four days after finishing #1 before you begin #2. Waiting periods are always beneficial

2. Calcarea Carb 30th potency—two pellets, three times a day for three days. Wait two-four days before taking #3

3. Lycopodium 30th potency— two pellets, three times a day for three days. Wait two-four days before #4

4. Sulphur 30th potency— two pellets, three times a day for three days.

5. Calc Phos 6X—one pellet (made by Hyland's, Tissue Cell Salt #2), three times a day for at least a month.

More details on this program

If for any reason, you do not complete the three-day dosing period for any of these remedies, and there is a gap of more than 24 hours since the last dose, do not attempt to go back and make up the difference. Just continue to the next remedy.

This is done because homeopathic remedies are an energy impulse to the energy bodies and follow different rules from material medicine. If an energy impulse was begun with a few doses then interrupted by a period of time (more than 24 hours between doses), DO NOT CONTINUE WITH THAT REMEDY. Beginning again will cause a clash of energy impulses and antidote the effect of the remedy.

If only one dose is missed, proceed with the same remedy to complete the three-day-dosing cycle. It is okay to crowd doses up at the end of the day.

Proper order of the Program:

NOTE:

- *Marking your calendar is a good way to make sure you don't forget or confuse the steps.*
- *Remedies in 30th potency can be either 30X or 30C but the "30" is essential.*
- *When a wait-period is called for, it is best to wait a few days to give time for the remedy to work on its own. This can be two to four days depending on what you feel is right for you.*

Week 1

Natrum Mur. 30th

Natrum Muriaticum is the first remedy because many people with old or unrecognized grief issues may have a dryness in the bones that prevents calcium from absorbing correctly. Natrum Mur. can put moisture back in bones and aid the absorption of calcium.

Take the remedy in a 2-pellet-dose under the tongue, three times a day for three days.

At the completion of this three-day-period, stop taking it.

Wait two to four days before continuing to the next remedy (see Note above). If you are anxious to go on, wait only two days. If you are experiencing positive changes in the way you feel and think, wait four days before continuing on to complete a full week's time. A wait time between remedies is always good.

Week 2

Calcarea Carbonica 30

Take three doses a day for three days only and wait a few days (see Note above). This is calcium carbonate already converted to energy to open receptor sites on cells to accept the calcium molecule.

Week 3

Lycopodium Clavatum 30

Take three doses (two pellets) a day for three days only and wait a few days (see Note above).

Lycopodium is a remedy from the plant kingdom that helps to hold the new receptor sites open to continue to absorb calcium.

Week 4

Sulphur 30

Be careful to buy Sulphur, no other word should be there (not Sulphur Iodatum or Sulphur Acidum) Take three doses (two pellets) a day for three days only. Wait a few days (see Note above).

This is elemental sulfur, a necessary nutrient that is often lacking where calcium absorption is low. This remedy allows sulfur to be absorbed into cells along with calcium.

Weeks 5 through 9

Calc. Phos. 6X

Take one pellet as a dose (made by Hyland's, Tissue Cell Salt #2), three doses a day for a period of at least a month.

The 6X potency works on the innermost energy bodies ensuring continued calcium absorption into deep internal layers of your body.

If you are very calcium deficient, you may want to continue to take Calc. Phos 6X for months, or as long as you feel changes occurring in your muscle tone.

Taking a calcium supplement at the same time you are on the Calc. Phos. 6X is appropriate. Any supplement product made by a reputable company, in a dosage of around 500mg taken once a day is good.

Do not overdose on calcium by taking 2000mg. It won't help.

Take calcium with food, since it needs stomach acid to break it down into usable components. Choose a supplement that also contains magnesium—magnesium and calcium are always absorbed together. Boron or Vitamin D included in the calcium supplement is okay, but it is best to avoid a product that includes zinc. Zinc can accumulate in tissue and cause toxicity.

If you continue to take a calcium supplement even after completing your month-long-regime with Calc. Phos. 6X, you should take a dose at least once a day. Taking the dose just before sleep will have the added benefit of helping you sleep. Calc Phos. 6X can be taken for a long time—even for a few years if you continue to see benefits.

Old Infections Aggravate

After you have taken calcium absorption remedies along with calcium supplements for a few weeks it is common to feel pain and old symptoms in areas where you have had a past infection. If this happens, know that these symptoms are normal and not a sign that the remedy isn't working.

A former client reported having chills and a feverish feeling accompanied by tightness in her chest. The symptoms disappeared after twelve hours but she was concerned about why it had happened. I explained that the absorption of calcium into her cells where the old infection occurred helped her immune system get rid of the remnants of the infection once and for all. She confirmed that she had had a life-long problem with upper-respiratory infections.

I have seen this aggravation of old pain in many of my clients who were using this program.

The aggravation of old infections can be painful and even frightening. If these are caused by the infusion of calcium into tissue where infection has occurred in the past, it will be temporary. **However, do not hesitate to see a doctor if the pain is severe, accompanied by fever, or lasts for more than 24 hours**.

If what you are experiencing is a new infection instead of an aggravation, the symptoms will get worse and will not subside within 24 hours. Definitely see a doctor if this is the case. Untreated infection can lead to permanent damage.

"Complementary therapies, like homeopathy, get to the cause - rather than just treating the symptoms......I know from my own experience that they work...I'd like to see doctors prescribing homeopathic treatment...."

—Peter Hain, Secretary of State, Wales, UK

Chapter 11
Metabolic Syndrome

- Have you been on a diet your entire life?

- Have you used stimulants to raise your metabolism and diet drinks to cut calories?

- Have you tried every diet that was ever invented and gained more weight after every one?

- Are you unable to stick to a diet because your body reacts badly every time you try and you end up gaining back more than you've lost?

Stimulants and diet drinks are the two diet aides that actually cause a person to gain weight.

Syndrome X

Metabolic Syndrome or "Syndrome X" is a condition in which your body becomes resistant to insulin. If you are insulin resistant, you are pre-diabetic and in danger of developing Type 2 Diabetes.

Common signs are a waistline over 35 inches in women and 40 inches in men, a fasting blood sugar level over 100mg/100mL, and a difficulty in losing weight.

This situation arises as insulin receptor sites on your cells stop functioning. Receptor sites are supposed to open in order to take in nutrients brought to the cell surface in the blood. In insulin resistance, the number of functioning receptor sites become reduced in number.

Medical research has revealed that obese people have interrupted insulin signaling pathways. These pathways are your body's bio-mechanisms designed to take insulin and glucose to the surface of individual cells. If glucose makes its way to a cell wall, it has a chance of being absorbed and used for energy. In obese people, a lot of the insulin and glucose never make it to the cells. Instead, the insulin and glucose are left to wander around and deposit in places they shouldn't, such as the liver, internal organs, the skin and the extremities.

This situation results in weight gain in the middle of the body, since your body has to store the excess insulin and glucose somewhere quickly and this part of the body is an easy target.

This condition is known as "Insulin Resistance" because the insulin is giving proper signals for sugar distribution, but your body isn't paying attention—it resists the commands of the insulin and direction is lost.

This would be similar to a freeway system with no signs to

direct the motorists. No one would know where to go.

In this condition, your cells don't get as much glucose as they need. These poor cells get hungry and send signals of hunger to your brain, which causes you to eat more—usually sugary or fatty foods because some of the fat and sugar calories do make their way to the cell walls.

Your appetite remains high because the cells are still unfed. Attempts to lose weight by skipping meals are undermined by the liver, which throws out excess glucose to feed the cells because the liver perceives that starvation is the reason for all of this chaos. The cells use the glucose delivered by the liver instead of metabolizing it from stored fat. Eventually, your body shuts down insulin production, resulting in obesity and eventually in diabetes.

Where did it all go so wrong?

What came first?

Did the initial weight gain cause the insulin signaling pathways to become interrupted or did other factors cause the direction malfunction that resulted in weight gain? Personally, I know my greatest weight gain began with the use of amphetamine drugs and diet drinks while in high school.

Diet Drinks Corrupt

I know that a lifetime of dieting caused many of my health problems, but it took time and contemplation to discover the mechanism of the weight-gain that is the symptom of deeper functional problems.

It has always seemed logical that if we cut calorie intake, we can reduce weight. However, only recently has it been found that a drink that tastes sweet, but does not contain calories actually works against our body by interrupting insulin-signaling pathways and shutting down receptor sites on cells.

After several months or years of consuming such beverages, particularly if no other nutrients are consumed at the same time, enough nutrient absorption has been interrupted that weight gain is inevitable.

The effect of this is that most calories taken in have to be stored. This starves our cells and they send messages to the brain calling for more nutrients. This increases hunger. The cycle of overeating and weight gain continues to accelerate.

This happens because our body does not know the difference between something that tastes sweet and has sugar and calories and nutrients and something that tastes sweet but has no calories or nutrients.

If you consume a sugar-free diet drink, the brain thinks that since it tastes sweet, there must be sugar present and sends a signal to the pancreas that sugar is on the way.

Since sugar needs insulin to enter into our cells, the pancreas responds by releasing insulin to break up the sugar and transfer it to the proper place.

With sugar-free drinks (and other artificially sweetened drinks and foods) the insulin reaches the blood stream but there is no sugar.

Insulin is then delivered to cells without sugar. The cells can't take in insulin without sugar attached, so they close some of their receptor sites to keep the insulin out. The insulin must be turned off with an insulin-inhibiting hormone and stored somewhere else, most likely in adipose tissue of the abdomen. The pathway to storage causes confusion for the body and normal pathways are corrupted.

Fat cells in the abdomen are not supposed to have this stored insulin combined with the insulin-inhibiting hormone. They begin to leak fats, which then find their way to the liver and other organs causing even more problems.

Eventually, the pancreas cuts back on insulin production because there is too much insulin in the bloodstream. At this point, we are in danger of developing type 2 diabetes. Eventually, insulin production stops all together and we can become an insulin-dependent diabetic.

During this process, sugar molecules that should have gone into cells are stored in the stomach and extremities along with a hormone that shuts down the effect of insulin. Blood vessels start to break down because of sugar stored in the muscle-tissue-layers in the veins—and the stored sugar causes inflammation that weakens veins. Cholesterol levels rise to settle down the inflammation and shore up rips in the blood vessels. Blood pressure is raised along with blood sugar and cholesterol levels.

After years of this situation, our body has stored enough sugar in the skin, internal organs and the extremities to begin compromising circulation and produce nerve pain.

This is where I found myself at the time I first experimented with the Gold Formula that I have developed. Right away I felt my body changing for the better.

Stimulants and fat-burners

Stimulating drugs and fat-burning herbal products cause the same receptor site shut-down and insulin resistance that diet drinks cause. Any stimulating product that we use to lose weight will contribute to obesity.

In the case of stimulants, our cells take in these substances and will, in the short-term raise our metabolism resulting in some weight loss. Over time, however, our cells cannot handle the stimulating effect and will close off receptor sites to keep the substance from entering.

After months or years of using these products, body weight will increase, seemingly without overeating. This excess weight includes a lot of belly fat.

Stimulants that could have contributed to this problem stretch back to the amphetamine culture of the 1960's. I was a part of that one. For four years, while I was in high school, I was given amphetamines by a doctor. Not only was any weight-loss temporary, but after those years, I gained my weight back, plus much more.

Every stimulant I took to lose weight, whether herbal or pharmaceutical, preceded another weight-gain-period in my life.

Other dangerous stimulants include: ephedrine, ephedra-based-products, pseudo-ephedrine and Ma Huang—the Chinese name for ephedrine.

Ginseng is another stimulant that will cause weight gain in many people. Some say that Chinese body builders and martial artists use this without a problem. That may be true, but those of us who have the weight-accumulating problem of receptor site shutdown will find that Ginseng contributes to weight gain.

Turin is a stimulant found in the energy drinks many people consume. Turin also contributes to obesity.

Any product that advertises energy-boosting effects will cause weight gain—not right away, but it will happen. When it does, it is almost impossible to reverse.

The weight-gain-effects of these products is so subtle and happens so slowly over time that it is difficult to realize exactly what takes place on the cellular level to cause the problem. However, if you look back over the history of your body's accumulation of bulk, you may find a connection to the times in your life when you either used one of these stimulants, or indulged heavily in diet soda or artificial sweeteners as a calorie control strategy—and that includes using Stevia as an artificial sweetener.

Emotion as a stimulant

Are diet sodas, stimulants, and such the only contributor to this kind of weight gain? No. About 1 percent of the population in the United States never or rarely used these diet strategies yet find themselves in the category of obese. This group accounts for the 1% of the population that was overweight before the diet craze caused the epidemic.

For these people, the offending substances are naturally occurring chemicals in the body that are produced during high levels of emotional stress.

The Role of Stress on Weight Gain

Just as with stimulants, a highly-charged emotional event, long-standing levels of stress or extreme grief will produce an over-abundance of lactic acid in the muscles that enters the blood stream and gets delivered to body cells. When cells cannot handle this excess of lactic acid, they shut down receptor sites to keep it out. Many people who become type 2 diabetics rather suddenly can often report an emotional or grief event that preceded the onset of the diabetic condition.

Toxicity Clearing

How does a homeopathic remedy based on metallic gold address the above problems?

Although there have yet been no scientific studies of the effects of this remedy, my experience has shown that our cells welcome the energy impulse of potentized gold and appear to open receptor sites to take it in.

People who have corrupted their insulin-signaling pathways by using diet drinks, energy drinks, and/or stimulants to lose weight and have accumulated a lot of weight over the years often find that weight-loss becomes possible when using a proper diet and exercise program.

Taking the gold-based remedy seems to aid a weight-loss

program when nothing worked prior to taking the formula. This is a strong indication that receptors sites that have been shut down due to insulin resistance may be starting to reopen.

As cells begin to absorb the energy signature of the gold, toxic residue from the inside of cells gets released.

When receptor sites open and toxins are released from cells into the blood stream, we experience an increase of toxicity through the digestive tract. This can create stomach symptoms as our body tries to eliminate these chemicals from the blood.

If you experience nausea, headache with dizziness, stomachache or diarrhea when beginning the Gold Formula, it is a sign that your body's toxin load is high. In order to release the toxins, you can take homeopathic Nux Vomica in a 30th potency until the symptoms subside, usually three days. If symptoms return, the frequency of taking the Gold remedy can be reduced and alternated with homeopathic Cocculus in a 6th potency to remove the toxins from your body until the gold can be taken without discomfort.

More Problems

Conventional efforts to fix a weight problem actually contribute to the problem. Stomach stapling surgery does not correct the cell-function problems that led to weight gain and causes many people who have gone that route to gain the weight back.

Regaining weight after a vigorous diet regime is one of the most heart-breaking experiences a person can go through, but it will continue to happen until the body can function properly to control weight naturally.

Arrest the Problem

Stop drinking diet sodas and artificially sweetened drinks, or use them only while eating a meal.

Don't use any stimulate to help in weight loss—including energy drinks. Coffee does not seem to affect the receptor sites if the amount consumed on a daily basis is less than 3 to 4 cups drunk throughout the day. Avoid putting saccharine or any other artificial sweetener in your coffee or iced tea.

Do the remedy program in Chapter 10. The use of the calcium absorption remedies helps to open up new receptor sites in the cells to receive calcium, which remain open to receive glucose from insulin, thereby increasing nutrient absorption into cells dramatically.

The Gold Formula is also helpful for restoring insulin-signaling pathways. Doing the calcium regime first and then following that with the Gold Formula is best.

NOTE: At the time of the publishing of this book, the Gold Formula is only available by contacting me directly.

Diet Virgins

If you are a diet virgin—someone who has never dieted before—you are unlikely to have a problem with insulin resistance unless you have been under stress for a long period of time, have had trouble sleeping for an extended period, grew up drinking energy drinks, or have suffered a major emotional event.

If have never dieted, it is likely that you have not created a body response that leads to a shut down of receptor sites. It may be easier to lose weight because your body does not yet know what is to come. You could probably use any diet and lose weight.

It is usually a diet virgin who becomes the poster child for new diet-aid products. Diet virgins are usually those who lose weight without any problem and keep it off. We were all able to do that in the beginning.

However, as time, stress, emotion, and failed diets jade your body against dieting and increases insulin resistance, no diet will work. Keep this in mind when you hear ads for the next great diet plan or product.

What is never really addressed is that most of us are not diet virgins and do not lose weight on any of these products, but the manufacturers want us to think we can. Most of us are diet junkies and none of these diets or products will work for us in actually creating weight loss.

If you are a diet junkie, you may have developed problems with the programs listed below.

Weight-Loss Problem

Many people who have lost a lot of weight on any diet program may experience gall bladder problems. Some have actually had their gall bladder surgically removed because of the pain that developed while on or after following a rigorous diet. The source of gall-bladder problems after losing weight is hard to pinpoint. But perhaps toxins and cholesterol coming out of fat cells and passing through the liver or being converted to bile, will clog the gall bladder with stones. Many times the pellet-like stones found in the gall bladder are composed of hardened cholesterol. Perhaps a low-fat diet can allow bile to remain in the gall bladder too long and cause stones to form.

If you have lost a lot of weight recently, or tried a low-fat diet, and you still have your gall bladder, but have some minor pain in the region, there is help. Gall bladder pain in its mildest form will be experienced as a pain or discomfort under the right scapular bone, or the right shoulder blade.

Sometimes this pain is so mild the sufferer will describe it as a tired feeling and attribute it to fatigue. However, it is most often mild radiated pain from the gall bladder. More severe pain will be actual pain on the right side of the abdomen above or at the waist—not to be confused with appendix pain in the low right abdomen.

IMPORTANT: If this pain is severe, do not hesitate to see a doctor. If this problem continues for too long untreated, the tissue of the gall bladder could begin causing serious complications. The homeopathic remedy suggested here is for reversal of a mild problem at a point at which the problem can be reversed. The pop artist Andy Warhol actually lost his life due to neglected gall bladder disease. This is not a condition to take lightly.

Formula for Reversing Mild Gall Bladder Condition

If your discomfort is mild and you want to try to reverse the condition, the remedy is:

- Cinchona Officionalis (common name is China, or Peruvian Bark) in a 30 X or C potency, taken three times a day for three days only.

- This is followed with Chelidonium Majus in the mother tincture, written as MT or Tincture. Put 7 to 10 drops in an ounce of water and drink the water three times a day for a period of one month.

Other remedies that help the gall bladder heal **after** completing the first two remedies are Aurum Met. 6X and Carbo Veg 6X.

These two remedies can be taken in alternating doses through the day. For example, take one pellet of the Aurum Met. remedy in the morning after breakfast then one pellet of the Carbo Veg. after lunch. One pellet of Aurum Met. in the early evening and one pellet of Carbo Veg in the late evening.

This can be done each day until the pain is gone, or can be continued for up to one month.

The High Fat, Low Carbohydrate Diet

Eliminating carbohydrates from your diet is a dangerous prospect. Symptoms your body will produce could include bloating, constipation, water retention, fogginess, gall bladder stones, kidney pain and possibly kidney stones.

Carbohydrates are necessary for normal body and brain function. Reducing carbohydrates may be okay for a short period of time, and may actually produce weight loss, but in the long-term, it can be dangerous. Any weight lost is usually regained quickly.

High protein can also inhibit calcium absorption causing kidney stones to form.

The remedy to help relieve kidney stress is Lycopodium, 30th potency, three times a day for three days, followed by Kali Phos. 6X for a month after.

This is general advice to eliminate any problem that may have arisen—even problems that you are not aware of, in order to eliminate the stress low-carb dieting may have caused to your system.

The Calcarea remedy of the program in Chapter 10 will also help eliminate the excess calcium associated with the possible formation of kidney stones.

IMPORTANT: If the problem is severe, and there is pain, do not hesitate to see a doctor. Kidney stones can be a life-threatening situation and should not be ignored.

Stomach Surgery

Those who have gone through the surgical procedure to staple their stomach and eliminate the capacity for large amounts of food in order to correct morbid obesity may find that after some time the weight starts to return.

This is because the underlying problem of calcium malabsorption and insulin resistance that caused the problem in the first place has not changed. Your body cells will still be unable to absorb calcium.

The calcium absorption program in Chapter 10 will help balance the problem. Zinc drainage will help eliminate excess zinc that has been liberated through fat loss, and it will stop your body's need to dilute zinc concentration with new weight gain (look in Chapter 19 for zinc drainage).

Vegetarianism

Vegetarian and vegan diets are difficult to balance for protein needs. They are also sometimes low in fat, which can be a problem. Many people on unbalanced vegetarian diets often have difficulty healing after injury. Most of this is due to the deficiency of amino acids, which are necessary nutrients found naturally in animal proteins.

One meal of chicken a week would help relieve some of these symptoms. For those who will not eat animal protein of any kind, amino acids in supplement form may help, but this is not the ideal solution. Taking a protein supplement may also be helpful.

Any diet that eliminates a particular food group is not good for the human body. In order to stay healthy, you cannot eliminate meat, carbohydrates, fats, or sugars.

In spite of best intentions or a desire to compensate kindness for cruelty to another living species, the reality is that human beings possess an omnivore, animal body. We cannot go against our natural need for proper nutrients and remain healthy.

Recognize the New You

After losing a lot of weight, you may look in the mirror one day and feel as if you are a completely different person than you used to be before the weight loss. This might be empowering, but it might also trigger a subconscious fear response that has you going on a campaign to regain the person you used to be.

To remedy this, a single dose of the homeopathic potentized form of Valerian Root, Valeriana in a 1M or 1,000th potency will help you recognize the new person you have become and feel comfortable with your new self image. This single dose can be repeated from time to time as weight is lost over a long period

---

Chapter 12

Grief and Sodium

When I worked at Capitol Drugs, a customer came in and told me that she was having trouble sleeping, had no appetite, and felt depressed. She also described a general achiness all over her body.

I asked her if there had been a grief situation lately. I wasn't prepared for her reaction.

She gasped, put her hands to her face, turned away from the counter, and burst into tears.

I quietly waited for her to compose herself. When she was ready, she told me that her baby had died at birth. She was heartbroken and angry at the world.

I asked if she had begun to crave salty foods. She answered yes, that chips had become a mainstay of her diet, which wasn't normal since she had always eaten healthy foods before.

I asked if she felt that every day was the same day as the tragedy and if she was having trouble getting on with her life.

She answered yes and described how depressed she was because she couldn't feel anything, couldn't think about anything other than how sad she was.

I suggested two remedies: Ignatia in a 30th potency to be taken for three days, and also Natrum Mur. 30C, to be taken for the next three days after the first remedy.

She called me about a year later to say that she had given birth to a healthy baby girl and life was great.

Ignatia is a universal homeopathic remedy. A universal remedy is a one that works for anyone in the same way, regardless of constitutional makeup.

Ignatia clears the effect of grief from the energy bodies and works for everyone in the same way no matter the situation. Anytime there is grief, from major to minor—a three-day course of Ignatia in a 30th

A universal remedy is a one that works for anyone in the same way, regardless of constitutional makeup.

potency is a useful remedy because grief can stay stuck in your energy body like a hard-shell-bubble that forces energy to flow around it. This can cause problems ranging anywhere from a sore throat to foot pain to depression to mania.

Sodium chloride is the chemical that our brain uses to process and put information into memory files. Grief can cause a sodium deficiency because the brain requires lots of it to process major grief.

If your body cannot deliver enough sodium, your brain cannot process information and you will feel as if you cannot get past that day your grief occurred. Even in the mildest of grief situations, there is often a sudden craving for salty food.

The craving is the result of the brain's demand for salt for the filing process—but the craving also indicates that the sodium isn't getting across into brain cells.

Your body will demand more salt by creating a craving because your brain cells are not getting what they need. Somehow, proper sodium absorption is blocked. As you eat more salt to satisfy your craving, blood pressure can rise as more sodium in the blood draws fluid from tissues.

By taking the homeopathic form of sodium, Natrum Muriaticum, the barrier that kept *Sometimes salt craving can be related to a situation so remote you can't remember why you are eating so much salt.* sodium from being absorbed is broken, sodium gets into cells as it should, craving goes away, grief is put into files as it should and you feel better.

The pain that caused the grief is never forgotten, just handled properly so that you can resume a normal life.

Sometimes salt craving can be related to a situation so remote you can't remember why you are eating so much salt.

I had a client who carried a little bag of rock salt in her purse to nibble on. She began to eat it while we were talking about her constitutional symptoms. I asked what she was eating. She said,

"Rock salt, umm, it's so good."

I immediately wrote Natrum Mur. 30C for her first remedy. The next time she came to the office I asked about her salt-eating-habit. She gave me a stunned look and smiled. "Oh, I had forgotten I used to do that."

Sodium Absorption Problems

It seems strange that so many people crave something so potentially harmful. Yet when homeopathic principles are understood, the explanation becomes surprisingly clear. Individual cells are not getting the sodium chloride they need. There is a block to cell absorption. The cells cry out for sodium because they can't get it. All the salt you eat sits in your intercellular fluid, piling up and causing problems such as dehydration, a decrease in spinal fluid, and high pressure in the blood vessels due to the attraction of fluid from tissue into the high sodium concentration flowing in the vessels.

I treated a four-year-old boy who was whinny, pale, thin and unable to speak clearly. He had been diagnosed by his doctor as anemic. He spoke only two words at a time, and even those were not easily understood.

I gave him a three-day-course of Nat. Mur in the 30th potency and four weeks later, I saw a lively, happy, playful boy. He was no longer thin, pale, sickly—and according to his doctor—no longer anemic. He was speaking better and using words more clearly. It was hard to believe he was the same child.

Anemia is a problem for sodium deficient people because

their bones will lack proper moisture.

Dry, brittle bones may not produce marrow that can correctly form red blood cells. These blood cells may not be able to carry enough iron and hemoglobin, leading to anemia. Often the problem is not the lack of iron but rather the inability of blood cells to carry enough of it.

Insufficient sodium absorption can also cause bones to be brittle. If bones are dry and brittle, calcium cannot absorb in sufficient amounts. That is why I put Natrum Mur. first in the calcium absorption program.

I treated a six-month-old baby who had fallen from his bed and snapped his leg.

I was astounded. A baby should not have bones brittle enough to break so easily. It seemed obvious to me he had a sodium absorption issue that manifested as a bone calcium problem, which would translate to other more difficult problems as he grew.

The Sodium Constitution

If you are someone who needs to balance sodium, a Natrum Mur. constitution, you will crave salty foods and add a lot of salt to your food or have a desire to add salt even if you have been told not to.

You will be thirsty, because your body is trying to put moisture in the places where it is needed, but it does not go where it should and can accumulate where it shouldn't.

This excess moisture can be in the form of edema—what

used to be called dropsy. You may even have high blood pressure due to the amount of sodium and fluid in your blood, yet your bones and brain tissue will go without and your bones become dry and brittle.

You might be anemic, since lack of moisture in your long bones—where the marrow is producing red blood cells—makes it difficult for marrow to produce blood cells correctly.

The mind of a Natrum Mur. constitution has problems processing information and keeping memory intact due to the lack of sodium. Sodium chloride as a chemical in brain tissue helps the brain process information and put that information into files to make it available for memory.

Without proper amounts of that chemical, your system malfunctions. If you are someone with a sodium constitution, you may have a life-long problem with learning disabilities. You might have been a student with noticeable difficulties learning to read, hated school, and avoided going to college.

Sometimes this symptom is subtle. Someone with this constitution might not read for pleasure because it is not easy or enjoyable and yet managed to graduate from college with a professional degree. This is likely a student who had to spend a lot of time studying compared to others who found reading easier and remembered the information effortlessly.

Children with a salt craving will have a problem learning to read, assimilating and processing what they read, and will probably hate school. Natrum Mur. remedies will make dramatic, positive changes for these kids.

Sodium Constitution and Grief

Many people are born with a sodium absorption problem, but it can also be acquired through extreme grief. Grief is an emotion that interferes with sodium absorption. Many people who have experienced grief, or a highly emotional situation, will suddenly become salt cravers. From that point on, the brain will not be able to process information correctly and the person loses interest in life or studies. They may develop headaches from eyestrain, begin to have trouble relating to people, and eventually will develop anemia or high blood pressure. The longer this situation goes on the more severe it becomes.

The accumulation of grief over a lifetime intensifies all of these problems, which manifests as the common symptoms and age related weakness and senility—which is wrongly considered normal. It doesn't have to be that way.

When given the sodium remedies, you will stop craving salt, your mind can process grief and you can go on with your life.

Communication Problems

I had a long-term client tell me about her twenty-two-year-old son who just stopped talking. He was completely normal through high school and had been attending college until he had dropped out to follow a girl he was in love with.

This young man had been involved in a religious group whose members attacked his character then expelled him. He not only lost membership in the group, he also lost close friends and his girlfriend.

His mother was relieved he had left the group, but concerned that he would not speak about it—and that he would not speak at all. His father was about to admit him to a mental hospital.

A few days later, she brought her son to the office. He didn't look odd or anti-social, and was not defiant in his demeanor. He appeared normal.

I asked him a question. He opened his mouth to speak, but nothing came out. He raised his hand in question and shook his head.

I asked him why he couldn't speak. He took out a piece of paper and wrote that he knew what he wanted to say, but couldn't get his mouth to say the words.

For this young man, his brain's ability to stimulate nerve responses to form speech had been interrupted by grief and a depletion of sodium. I gave him a single dose of Natrum Mur. 10M.

About three weeks later I got a phone call. The mother put her son on the line to talk to me. His ability to speak had completely returned to normal.

In this situation, the intense level of grief he had experienced caused sodium depletion in brain tissue causing symptoms that had not existed before.

Chapter 13
Mental Injury

Fear

Fear takes many forms. One is displayed by those who stay in jobs they hate, still live in towns where they grew up, or in the house they lived in for decades because of a fear of leaving their routine and trying something different.

Most of these people are miserable and want more out of life but are not aware of why they fail to try. Arsenicum Album in a 30th potency is a remedy that helps eliminate this sort of fear.

Paranoid Fear

For those gripped by paranoid fear, there is a need to be in control at all times. They must constantly attempt to feel safe by making sure they are in control of their lives, other people's lives, and everything in their life arena.

These people may appear powerful—and may be powerful in certain contexts. However, they are often unapproachable, unlovable and unable to form lasting relationships. They have to make sure no one comes close enough to cause them harm.

This type of fear is most often learned as a small child—usually before they were old enough to understand the manipulation of care-giving adults. This fearful reaction is often seen in someone who was subjected to hospitalization as an infant. If an individual suffered traumatic injury, major surgery, major illness, or long separation from the birth mother for any reason, some degree of fearful behavior is to be expected.

Most people who have this issue are unaware of it. Kali Bromatum in a single 1M potency dose helps to clear this problem homeopathically.

Physical Fear

Still another form of fear is physical and can be the result of an injury that has left the sufferer dazed and confused, with headaches, anxiety attacks, and difficult or shallow breathing.

This fear causes heart palpitations, flushing, and fear of people, thunder, lightening, the nighttime, or a knock on the door. The fear could have originated with a back injury, whiplash, spinal administered medication, or minor blows to the spinal area. This type of fear is the result of an interruption in spinal-fluid flow. The fluid around the brain is less than it should be and fearfulness is the result.

I have seen this symptom in children who carry large, heavy

backpacks to school. The bag impacts the spine while the child walks, plays, or runs. The result can be night terrors, insomnia, or a generalized fearfulness. The remedy is Aconitum Nap. taken in a 30th potency three times a day for three days—and only three days—to relieve the symptoms, followed with Natrum Mur. 6X for a month to put moisture back in the spinal column.

The Formation of Anger

If something occurred in your life that made you feel worthless, there will be physical changes. These changes can be from being shamed by another person trying to make him/herself appear powerful.

This sort of shaming can be by a parent, sibling, classmate, or spouse. It can also be the result of crime victimization. Whatever the cause, this experience always results in deep-seated anger—so deep it can be felt physically.

Those who have suffered this kind of trauma react to most things in their life with an anger response.

Anger can cloud their entire life and impact every aspect of it. This pain can hurt so much the sufferer doesn't want to live. They will either numb themselves with alcohol or drugs, or disengaging the energy bodies. There can be just enough blurring of the lines of connectedness between the body and the soul to dull the pain sensations. The conscious mind would be totally unaware that this has occurred.

When this disconnectedness happens, feelings of hunger, fullness, physical pain, love or pleasure are numbed. This can cause obsessive eating because the sufferer has no idea when their body needs nourishment, has had too much food, or when it is suffering from the effects of over indulgence.

Others may describe this person as "dead inside." They are unable to cry, feel sadness, or express emotion.

These sufferers crave foods high in salt, such as chips, pretzels or cheese snacks because sodium absorption has been interrupted by the emotion, which causes an entire complex of problems.

Alfalfa in a 30th potency, taken three times a day for three days works wonders. Even if all of the above symptoms are not present, everyone could use a three-day-dosing of Alfalfa 30 at least once in their life because everyone probably harbors some level of anger.

Alfalfa is most often used as an energy tonic in homeopathic combination formulas. The 30th potency may be difficult to find because it has not been recognized as a remedy for anger. Look for it on line, any brand will work, but it must be a 30th potency, either 30C or 30X. If you take it, you will feel an immense calmness after the three-day-dosing of the 30th potency.

The Effects of Grief

Consider how you would feel if everything in your life were going great until suddenly something so profound happened you felt as though you could not continue living and every day felt the same as the day of the tragic event.

That is what profound grief feels like.

The early death of a loved one or an accident that takes a child are examples of events so traumatic they create this sort of grief. Sometimes it does not have to be so devastating an event. In extremely sensitive people, the loss of a job or a move to a new city will create a grief situation.

Profound grief injures the soul. I observed a lot of this in my regular clients after the 9/11 attacks on New York's Twin Towers and The Pentagon. Many people were so deeply shocked by what happened that they reacted with symptoms of profound grief—becoming fearful of going out of the house, insomnia, a ball sensation and tightening in the throat, feelings of sadness but not being able to talk about it.

If you cannot talk about anything but this tragic event and talk about it all the time, wherever you go, you are in need of the sodium absorption remedy, Natrum Mur. in a 1M potency, one dose only. If you don't want to talk about it and want everyone else to stop reminding you, take Ignatia Amara in a 30th potency, three times a day for three days.

Anyone who suffers an injury so profound it injures the soul will need Arnica Montana in a single 1M potency dose. This is particularly true if the event caused feelings of agoraphobia and you fear leaving the house. The 1M potency of Arnica is most appropriate because the injury to the soul impacts the higher energy levels. Agoraphobia develops when the trauma is not in the physical body, and not related to personal grief, but rather occurs with feelings of horror and empathy for others.

When left untreated, this kind of injury penetrates inward to the energy bodies and brings on fears of the outside world.

Natrum Mur. 1M and Arnica Montana 1M in a single dose each, taken one at a time and not together, can relieve all of these problems and return the person to full habitation of their body, allowing a full return to sensations such as hunger, satiation, sadness and happiness.

Math Ability

A common example of a brain chemistry problem that translates into what appears to be a social problem is an adolescent girl who stops being a good student at the age of 12 or 13 and begins to be interested in boys.

I have heard this situation described many times by parents and teachers. I have known teachers who knew female students in the fifth grade and described these girls as brilliant, straight-A students and very good at math but who lost these qualities when they entered the sixth grade.

What took place between the fifth and sixth grades to change these good students into girls who suddenly begin to notice boys?

Many educators believe it is a socialization problem at the time students are going through puberty and beginning to notice the opposite sex. But is it only?

What actually occurs at this age is the onset of the menstrual cycle. In many girls, particularly those with the disposition to be calcium deficient, the onset of the monthly menstrual cycle can mean that iron is lost through blood loss each month. It shouldn't be this way, but commonly is. As girls lose iron, the brain loses iron as a chemical necessary to do math and other calculating skills.

Boys mature more slowly and over a longer period of time. They never develop an iron-losing cycle and never lose an ability to do math if they had the skill in the earlier grades.

Using Ferrum Metallicum as a remedy in a 1M dose for mental development is a way to restore the ability to calculate math for anyone, who displays a problem in this area. This remedy dose stabilizes iron in brain tissue. Follow this with a mild multiple vitamin that contains iron or increase the amount of iron rich foods in the diet such as nuts and spinach. Repeat this regime from time to time as needed.

Self Esteem

Self-esteem problems may also appear as shyness. A person who is calcium and copper deficient has a very difficult time judging how they relate to other people. Many sufferers cannot read people and do not know if people like them, if what they say is appropriate, or even if people are laughing at them or not.

In this stage of uncertainty, it is much easier to avoid social situations than to try to understand how they actually relate to the world.

Calcium and copper in homeopathic forms can clear these problems, allowing the person to be all that they can be and achieve all that is possible for them to achieve.

If this is something you suffer from, there are two high potency calcium-absorption-based remedies to restore self-awareness. The first one is Baryta Carb. in a single 10M potency dose. This one must come first. After a few days or perhaps a week, the second remedy is Calcarea Silicata 10M in a single dose. They must be taken in this order, Baryta Carb. first, followed by Calcarea Silicata, and only one dose each. Wait a few weeks. If it's working, you will find that you rely less on other people for confirmation of your actions and ideas and more on your own judgment.

Homeopathic copper, Cuprum Metalicum, is a remedy that can actually create new brain cells. Taken in a 6x over a period of a month, it will begin to help you expand brain function by increasing brainpower.

However, it may feel just the opposite during the process. One sign that a person is copper deficient is if they seem allergic to melons and have an itchy throat sensation while eating cantaloupe or honeydew melons. Cuprum Met. in any potency will clear the symptom. Cuprum Met. 6x taken for a month, three times a day, will also help hyperactive kids to calm down. The remedy seems to increase brain function and attention span.

With the end of fear, shame, anger and grief and the opening of the mind to the higher purposes life can hold, it is possible for the individual to experience life as it was meant to be lived—with joy, understanding and inner confidence—this is Thothology in action.

Chapter 14
Mental Enhancement Potencies

The Mind

Some remedies for mental-enhancement do not depend on constitutional symptoms to be useful. These remedies can be used by anyone who desires to solve a mental problem, or to improve thinking ability. They can be used by anyone with symptoms of A.D.D., has experienced brain damage, or anyone who just wants to sharpen cognitive function.

High potency mental-enhancement remedies are taken in a single dose—only one—and not repeated for at least a year because many cognitive functions influenced by high-potency-remedies can take several months to fully develop and complete the work needed to change mental abilities.

If a remedy is repeated before the full developmental duration has been completed, there may an antidote effect. Once the remedy has completely developed, it will be permanent.

The remedy may be repeated after a year to take development to an even higher level. Potency for these remedies is usually a 1M or a 10M dose that works on the outermost energy bodies and levels, and has little or nothing to do with constitution. These remedies can be taken by anyone over the age of 8 years.

You should not take more than one of these 1M or 10M potencies in a single day. It is best to take different ones at a pace of about once a week.

If time for dosing is short, they may be taken once a day because they will cue up in your energy levels and wait their turn to work. A more reliable alternative, though, is to dose only once a week.

Expect some time to pass before noticing the changes. Because of how our self-awareness works, these types of changes are often first noticed by those around us before we become conscious of them.

Attention Deficit

This is a problem that affects both children and adults. Sometimes it is due to brain damage from birth trauma or jaundice shortly after birth. Sometimes the problem is a result of physical toxicity.

Remedies:

- Stramonium 10M to help the small eye muscles coordinate with the brain to accept information while reading.

- I have seen many people become perfectly comfortable

with reading where there was only frustration
and conflict before the remedy was taken.

- Avena Sativa 10M to widen the attention
span and help with studying.

- Argentum Nit. in a single 10M dose also improves
attention span. It is all right to use both, but they
should be in separate doses and at different times.

- Natrum Mur. 10M helps the nutrient absorption of
sodium chloride and open channels to learning by
increasing the brain's ability to form memories.

- Coffea Cruda 10M increases the power to think. If
coffee helps you get started in the morning, Coffea
Cruda 10M will improve thinking power permanently.

- Colchicum 10 M helps alleviate an aversion to
mental labor. A lot of mental labor and learning is
accompanied by the release of adrenalin. If you
were abused at some time in your past, adrenalin
may feel uncomfortable, which will cause learning
to feel uncomfortable. This could explain why
many abused children are poor learners.

- Guaiacum 10M is needed if you have a problem
knowing how pieces of information fit together
into a larger whole. The action of the potency
stretches information files in the brain. This
allows for information to be shared between
files—much as an Internet search engine.

- Tuberculinum 10M opens channels to understanding.

- Medorrhinum 10M helps improve memory.

The two remedies—Tuberculinum and Medorrhinum are Nosodes—remedies made from disease causing organisms. In homeopathy, the potentizing of a disease bacteria means the DNA structure of the original entity is energized for healing rather than a molecular structure, as in other remedies.

Because of a misunderstanding over the effect of potentizing, nosodes have been banned for sale to non-professional individuals in the United States by the FDA. This is due to a fear that the disease-causing-organism in the nosode could actually cause disease. I have successfully, effectively, and safely used nosodes for years without any ill effects. In fact, they are some of the easiest remedies to use because they rarely cause aggravations.

If you can get them, Tuberculinum and Medorrhinum are powerfully effective. Some homeopathic pharmacies will allow the sale of a nosode with the approval of a professional homeopath.

The Tuberculinum nosode is made from the bacteria that causes Tuberculosis. In a potentized, homeopathic form, it improves the ability to understand complex problems.

The Medorrhinum nosode is made from the Gonorrhea bacteria.

Perhaps, if an ancestor suffered from either of these two illnesses, which can cause damage to DNA, you could have inherited the damage, which could be corrected by the high potency remedy.

In a more general sense, these nosodes improve overall function of DNA.

The symptoms of manic/depressive disorder can be relieved by Tuberculinum used in a 30th potency, three times a day for three days. The 30th potency is the best potency because the manic/depressive disorder originates in the physical expression of DNA.

Because Tuberculinum is a DNA-based potentized remedy, it can change the physical expression of genetic material.

Tuberculinum may not be used to treat active Tuberculosis.

Anti-Social Behavior

If a child is not bonding with a parent or displays anti-social behavior such as not being able to take authority, shows rebelliousness, or a lack of ability to get along with others, and the child also craves either chocolate or vanilla, this behavior could be caused by an inability of the brain to hang onto certain chemicals.

If the child wants chocolate everyday, or craves vanilla ice cream—and exhibits anti-social behavior, a homeopathic remedy made from those common foods could help.

Craving is an indication of the brain's inability to hold onto the chemical that chocolate or vanilla releases into brain tissue while being ingested.

Giving Chocolate or Vanilla as a homeopathic remedy will stabilize the chemicals in the brain that can improve behavior.

The child's body has attempted to compensate for the dysfunction by creating a craving for these chemicals. In the case of Chocolate and Vanilla, the potency is a 30th potency three times a day for three days.

In the United States, these two food-based-remedies are difficult to find. One source at the time of this writing is abchomeopathy.com/shop.php

Self-Image

If something has happened that changed the shape or structure of your body, one result could be emotional distress over no longer recognizing who you are as a person.

A single dose of Lachesis 1M can help you become more emotionally comfortable with physical changes.

Have you ever been with someone who looked in a mirror and said, "I don't recognize myself any longer?"

If you've lost a lot of weight, you might feel confused and uncomfortable in your new body, especially if you've carried excess weight for most of your life. This feeling is often a contributing factor in regaining the weight you so painstakingly lost.

Valeriana, in a single 1M potency will help you recognize and accept your new self .

Indecisive and Unfocused-Wishy-Washy Thinking

Do you have difficulty making decisions or focusing on a particular subject long enough to learn or get something done? This is a condition I call wishy-washy thinking.

I recommend two remedies to change this.

Silicea 1M will help clear the stress chemicals that have led to indecisiveness.

IMPORTANT: Silicea cannot be used by anyone who has a replacement body part. This rule includes lenses embedded in the eyes, screws in bones, knee or hip replacement, or dental implants. Although, crowns and fillings on teeth are not a problem. Silicea in any potency has the potential to expel foreign objects from body tissue and bone. Silicea is not recommended for people who have had an organ transplant. Since the DNA of the new organ would be different than the DNA of the rest of the body, complications could arise.

- Gelsemium 1M can clear problems with making decisions when the cause has been damage from viruses or brain injury from disease.

- Hamamelis 1M potency can help with combative behavior that stems from a feeling of not being respected.

- Rheum 1M potency works to restore patience if impatience is so acute even starting new projects is too much to bear. This is common in young people.

- Digitalis 1M helps to open up new abilities in the brain.

For children below 8 years old, use a 200th because the outermost energy bodies and levels have not fully developed and the 1M potency will have no where to sit.

If you try some of these mental enhancement remedies, just remember that the effect can be fascinating, but take time to develop, so have patience.

Homeopathy is a highly developed health practice that uses a systematic approach to the totality of a person's health. Anyone seeking a fuller understanding of health and healing will find Homeopathy extremely important and applicable.

— Gay Gaer Luce, PhD. twice winner of the National Science Writer's Award.

Chapter 15
Acute Dosing and First Aide

Several homeopathic remedies are universal and work the same for everyone who takes them— no matter the state of health or the pattern of constitution. These universal remedies can be taken in doses of short duration to stop acute illness or to lessen the effect of injury.

Cold and Flu

As soon as you begin to feel the effects of a cold or the flu virus—when the throat is just beginning the feel scratchy or sore, when your body is just starting to feel achy, or a fever is about to bring on a headache, it is possible to throw the flu or cold virus out of the energy bodies my using a product call *Oscillococcinum®* made by the Boiron Company. *Oscillococcinum®* is sold in most online and retail stores that carry homeopathy.

Taking a dose of about 7 or 8 pellets, three times in a 12 hour-period can throw the virus out of your energy bodies and impulse the immune system to fight the invading virus before it gets a hold on your physical body.

If it does not work to completely eliminate the virus, it will help to lessen the effect and shorten the duration of the illness.

Sometimes it happens that your immune system does not recognize a virus at all and has no defense against it. In this situation, an illness will develop in spite of everything used to stop it.

If you continue to develop a cold or flu after using *Oscillococcinum®*, you may still have a chance to throw it off by using Aconitum Nap. in a 200 potency.

Take this remedy three times in one hour—once on the hour, once at the half-hour, and again on the hour.

This acute dosing style is effective in most cases to stop a flu or cold virus in its tracks. If you only have a 30th potency on hand, the same effect may be achieved by taking a dose of the 30th potency every 10 minutes for an hour or two.

Stop taking it when you begin to feel better.

Also, Zincum Met. 6X will help boost your immune system to help throw off the illness. Use Zincum Met. 6X after the one-hour-acute dosing of Aconitum Nap. is complete.

On the rare occasions when these three remedies have not stopped the flu or cold from developing because the immune system did not recognize the invading virus, it is possible to shorten the duration of the illness by alternating doses of Natrum Mur. with Arsenicum Album.

Keep a 30th potency of each of these remedies on hand for

this purpose. Take them in alternating doses every 10 minutes for an hour. After the first hour, take alternating doses of each, once an hour for the next 12 hours.

Once, when I was substitute teaching, the students in my classes started coming down with the flu. I knew it was only a matter of time before I caught it as well. This was just before the Christmas break and I had planned to travel out of town for the holidays. Of course, I started getting sick the night before my scheduled trip. I don't know where the idea came from—I guess it was just one of those intuitive moments—but I decided to try alternating acute doses of the two remedies. My theory was that the Arsenicum Album would stem the body's allergic reaction to the virus—which is the cause of all the miserable symptoms— and that the Natrum Mur. would remove any emotional reason why my immune system had failed to protect me.

I had a 200th potency of each. I dissolved a pellet of each remedy in separate bottles of water and alternated doses from each bottle by sipping the water about every half hour (bottle A then wait half hour and sip from bottle B, and so on) for the first few hours, then every hour for the entire nine-hour-trip.

During this dosing period I felt horrible. The flu symptoms were particularly bad—and I just felt retched. That night I slept really soundly and woke around 11:00AM feeling great. I had no flu symptoms. The remedies had completely driven the virus out of my energy bodies. I had a bit of lingering congestion, but nothing of the misery from the day before.

If, 24 hours after taking the remedies, you still have some

lingering symptoms, you can take Kali Bichromium for a stuffy runny nose. Pulsatilla if your nose is just runny. Antimonium Crude if you have chest congestion.

Regardless of remedies, see a medical professional if your symptoms are severe.

Build Your Immunity

Oscillococcinum® may be taken once a month as a preventative to viral infection, however, repeating it within the month after it was taken can antidote the effect. The dose is 9 or 10 pellets (the amount doesn't matter), three times within 12 hours.

Mark your calendar when you take your first dose. If you have taken *Oscillococcinum®* within that month and flu-like symptoms develop, do not repeat it. Instead, take other remedies for boosting your immune system against the flu. I recommend Zincum Met. and Aconitum Nap. 200 if symptoms continue to develop.

After taking *Oscillococcinum®* every month for a couple of years, you can just use it whenever you feel a possible flu or cold coming on. This may help you become immune to flu viruses.

Sudden Injury

Because there is always the possibility of sudden unexpected injury, it is wise to keep Arnica Montana on hand.

In the case of injury, take Arnica Montana in a 30th potency, every 10 minutes for up to 2 hours as soon as possible after an injury to lessen the severity and speed healing. If a 200th potency is available, take it every 10 minutes for one hour.

This style of dosing works to lessen the impact of the injury because injury causes damage over time as the impact penetrates through the energy bodies from the outside toward the internal. Before the full extent of the injury has penetrated all levels of the energy bodies, it is possible to throw the effect off of the outer most energy bodies and modify severity.

If your injury is severe enough to require stitches, surgery or casting, do not expect Arnica to offset the need for treatment. See a medical professional. Homeopathy cannot completely reverse that sort of damage to the physical body.

Arnica can offset the effect of bruising, relieve much of the pain, or stop swelling before it develops. However, seek medical aid as soon as possible when it is needed.

The use of Arnica can speed healing and shorten recovery after the medical procedure.

If you have a head injury, alternate Arnica Montana with any potency of Natrum Sulph. This remedy helps prevent swelling which can lead to concussion after head trauma.

Surgery

When using Arnica Montana, recovery time is often remarkable fast. This remedy increases your ability to heal and handle the changes your body endures during surgery. In order to prepare for surgery. begin two days before surgery and continue for five days after.

Take s of 2 pellets at a time in a 30th (either x or c) potency three times a day.

For healing wounds on your skin such as incisions, cuts and scrapes, use Calendula in the gel, cream and ointment form.

Pain

Homeopathic remedies do not have the same influence over the body that drugs do. They cannot block or overshadow pain, but one remedy, Hypericum Perf., can calm nerve endings to relieve some pain. Hypericum is usually taken 2 pellets at a time in a 30th (either x or c) potency three times a day for three days. Hypericum Perf. in the 6th potency can be taken long term for chronic pain. Take a dose of 1 to 2 pellets as needed.

Hypericum 30c is a good remedy to help heal damaged nerves. Alternate it with Salicylicum Acidum, 30th potency, at different times of the day—up to three doses a day of each, but only for three days.

Burns

Because the pure substance known as Cantharis can cause burns, in a homeopathic potency, Cantharis can help relieve the effects of a burn. Taken in a 30th potency, every 10 minutes for an hour, this remedy can lesson the severity of burns and cause the area of the skin affected to begin immediate healing.

A first-degree burn could disappear entirely with no redness or pain after a few doses. A second-degree burn could be prevented from blistering and pain decreased after several doses. A third-degree burn, however, will require treatment from a doctor, but the Cantharis will lesson severity and allow for quicker healing.

After the first hour, continue to take three doses a day for three days. I suggest keeping this remedy on hand.

Cantharis can also be helpful for sun exposure. For the best results, take the remedy as soon as possible after over-exposure to the sun. It is also possible to take preventive doses before spending a long period of time in the sun. It this case, one can take a 30th potency dose once every few hours during the day, increasing to short frequent doses as the time of exposure increases.

If you begin to feel dizzy, stop taking Cantharis immediately.

Eating Disorders

If you are not eating because you have an eating disorder, grieving, or are recovering from surgery, Zincum Metallicum in a 30th potency—one or two doses will help restore your appetite. I have seen anorexic teens return to healthy eating soon after taking their first dose of Zincum.

Dietary Zinc

Too much Zinc from supplementation can cause an increase in appetite as the body attempts to dilute the overload. Stop Zinc supplementation and use Zincum Met. 30th three times a day for three days to eliminate the excess.

Detox

Below are three common issues that are caused by a need to detox.

- **Nausea**

- If you suffer from nausea, suspected mild food poisoning, need to antidote or detox the effects of a drug, or to detox from anesthesia, take Nux Vomica in a 2-pellet-dose, 30th potency, three times a day for three days.

- **Morning Sickness**

- Carbo Veg. 6X or 6C, helps settle the stomach. Take a 2-pellet-dose as needed.

- **Motion Sickness**

- Cocculus 6X or 6C in a 2 pellet dose any time and as often as needed before and during the journey will relieve or prevent it.

Menopausal problems

A few years ago the results of studies made on hormone replacement therapy for menopausal women were released to the public. The use of hormones was found to increase the risk of heart disease and stroke. This was confusing since previously, the therapy had been recommended to reduce the risk of these two medical problems. Many women who did not intend to take replacement hormones had been persuaded to do so by their medical professionals with the promise they would be protected from future heart and blood vessel problems, leaving many dazed and disillusioned when they found that they still suffered the very symptoms the hormones were supposed to relieve.

It is my experience that most women who have problems during menopause usually find relief with the homeopathic remedy Sulphur—the nutrient responsible for the proper viscosity of body fluids. Being deficient in sulfur leads to night sweats, late-night sleeplessness, recurring sinus infections—all the usual symptoms associated with menopause.

To relieve these annoying symptoms, Sulphur 30, taken three times a day for three days, along with the nutritional supplement MSM (1000mgs), helps your cells absorb sulfur properly, thereby eliminating annoying symptoms.

Using the calcium and magnesium remedies in the program described in earlier chapters also helps eliminate other symptoms associated with menopause, such as osteoporosis, blood vessel integrity problems, heart disease symptoms—as well as migraine headaches due to hormonal imbalance that can occur or recur at menopause.

Homeopathy did not merely seek to cure
a disease but treated a disease as a sign of
disorder of the whole human organism. This was
also recognized in the Upanishad which spoke of
human organs as combination of body mind and
spirit. Homeopathy would pay an important part in
the Public Health of the country along with other
systems. Medical facilities in India are so scanty
that Homeopathy can confidently visualize a vast
field of expansion.

    –Dr. S. Radha Krishnan – Former President,
Govt. of India

Chapter 16

Autism

In recent years, I have worked with a large number of families with autistic children. Through this experience, I have discovered patterns that are common among individuals who suffer from this disorder.

Autism affects all ethnicities, economic groups and geographical locations. Some parents saw an onset of symptoms after a vaccine was administered. Some saw no relation to vaccines. Some children were never vaccinated at all. Some families have more than one autistic child.

There are two common factors in every family I have talked to—one is the presence of a member of the child's genetic line that is of genius-level intelligence. This is not necessarily an individual who has achieved great success or high levels of education, although those aspects may be present. The main benchmarks are extreme memory capability, mental processing speed and information gathering abilities.

The genius in the family is most often the child's father, but can also be the mother's father—in which case the mother is also of high intelligence. Sometimes there are multiple geniuses within the family. In all cases, the symptoms of autism flow from a member of the genetic line with advanced mental ability. Often, the geniuses in the family will display mild symptoms of autism spectrum disorders such as sensory sensitivity and awkward social skills.

The second common factor the parents report is that the symptoms of autism in their children developed at about the same time, between 16 and 18 months of age. This is the age when the 6th energy body should have begun to develop, but somehow didn't.

Because the formation of the energy bodies has stalled, the development of a complete energy level has also been arrested (revisit Chapter 2 to understand energy levels).

In my opinion, these children are inheriting a pre-disposition to highly advanced brainpower. My theory is that due to environmental factors, the child's mental-intelligence-level is even more advanced than the parent. So advanced in fact that the body is lacking the ability to deliver proper nutrients to fully express that brainpower.

The symptoms I see in these individuals are consistent with under-development of energy bodies and levels and include:

An unusually strong bond to a parent (the child does not perceive themselves as a separate individual and must be around a person with fully-functional energy bodies).

Extreme fearfulness or complete lack of fear (an inability to understand their surroundings).

Unawareness of time or the sequential nature of time (the energy level connection to time has not developed).

The inability to comprehend speech or produce speech (brain-files for language are underdeveloped as are the muscles to form speech).

Avoiding eye contact with people or keeping eyelids half-closed over pupils (limiting information input since processing of is slow).

Sound sensitivity (unable to process loud or intrusive sound such as in a crowd of people).

These symptoms are completely in line with the underdevelopment of energy bodies and levels.

The remedies that I have developed help the brain absorb the nutrients necessary to allow the energy bodies and mental energy level, and subsequent levels, to develop properly. This mineral-absorption-impulse and energy-level-development allows the child to understand and express language, become aware of their surroundings and understand how their behavior impacts other people.

What Autism Is Not

Autism is not a disease. Children displaying symptoms of autism spectrum disorders are not damaged. An autistic child is able to perceive energy beyond the conventional three-dimensional structure the rest of us live within.

The symptoms of autism are a reaction to changes in the global atmosphere. That is why the epidemic continues to deepen. For decades, metaphysical sources have been warning that these changes were coming. The first forewarnings began in 1987 at the time the outer most planets in our solar system first entered the Photon Belt. Since December of 2012, our entire solar system has been traveling through this Photon cloud full time. So, what does this mean?

The Photon Belt is a band of ionized particles emanating from the center of our galaxy. Our solar system passes through this belt every 13,000 years and takes about 2,000 years to traverse completely. As we enter the Age of Aquarius, our solar system is inside this cloud and inundated with these photon particles. When we are in the Photon Belt, human consciousness expands and the earth and her inhabitants undergo major changes.

The symptoms of autism are a reaction to changes in the global atmosphere. That is why the epidemic continues to deepen.

The problem this time is that there are 7 billion people on the planet. In their present physical condition, many people are not able to easily handle the changes that are taking place. Those who are not ready for the energy shift on the planet are feeling great stress without knowing why. This causes extremes in personal beliefs, erratic behavior and social upheaval.

It cannot be denied that the world is changing—from global warming to the human psyche—major changes are taking place.

For some time now, children have been born who have specialized abilities and are even physically unique. Metaphysically, it is believed that these children will somehow be instrumental in heralding in a golden age.

But there is a problem. The brains of these special individuals are not able to absorb the nutrients necessary to fully express all spectrums of the advanced multi-dimensional brainpower. Autism is a manifestation of this mineral-absorption-deficiency.

I've been working with homeopathic remedies and autistic individuals since 1982—before autism was an epidemic. The single remedy that cured the autistic brain early on was a simple solution.

Through the decades, the autistic kids I have worked with have changed. In the early years, many kids needed only one dose of a single remedy to begin developing normally. Later on, additional remedies were needed. However, the vibrational rate of information processing in the brain of the autistic children of today has become so advanced that an advanced set of remedies is necessary.

Recently, I have developed remedy formulas that are exactly what the autistic children need to help them expand their energy structures, perceive their surroundings and develop communication skills. With my remedy protocol, the child is able to form speech as well as retain savant abilities and intuitive genius. However, these changes do not take place without consequences. Many children experience emotional turmoil and behavioral aggravations during the course of the six-week-long protocol. This is particularly true for children on multiple-supplement therapies, which can create a battle between the chemicals in heavy supplementation and the body's attempts to heal the brain. Nevertheless, by the end of the treatment or shortly after, many kids experience great advancement in speech, conversational skills and awareness of their surroundings.

During and after the completion of the protocol remedies, the child's energy bodies begin to develop—as they should have at 18 months. But if the child is now 5 or 6 or even older, the development of those energy-body-based functions may seem chaotic and disturbing. It isn't always this way, but it can happen. This is because a particular behavior in a baby may be a minor occurrence and hardly worth noting. But at the age of 6 years, these behaviors can seem aggressive and not at all cute.

For example, all babies go through a chewing phase. This is not just for teething, but also for tone in the muscles of the face and mouth that will eventually produce speech. If the child is older and develops a chewing phase during or after the protocol is completed, this phase could seem aggressive and out of line, when in reality it is a normal part of development.

Perhaps the child has become stubborn or willful. This behavior is in line with the 'terrible two's' stage in a normal child. It is part of the brain and energy level development of awareness of the individual's place in the family and that they can manipulate their environment. But in a child of 7 or 8, this can seem excessive and difficult to deal with.

Every child is different. If you see some of these behaviors during or after the protocol, just know that it is part of the process of the child developing normal function.

The Genius

Autistic individuals are extremely intelligent. The moms I talk to know this and observe the genius through the symptoms. These kids perceive signs and signals the rest of us are clueless to. They see the world differently and perceive more clearly things 'normal' people don't.

We must recognize that even after recovery these children will be different. They may never go to standard institutions of higher education or enter conventional professions. But, what these individuals offer us is exactly what we will need in the future.

Just look at the past. Most of the great geniuses of history, the people who brought new, exciting innovations and thinking to the world, were often individuals who displayed many symptoms of what we now call autism. Included in this list are names such as Vincent Van Gogh, Michelangelo, Isaac Newton, Beethoven, and Einstein—and ever as far back as Socrates. The autistic genius has always been a part of mankind, but it has never before been as deep or as widespread as we find in the present day.

The Protocol

My protocol for autism takes 6 weeks to complete.

The remedies are based on necessary nutrients that are

blocked from being absorbed into the brain correctly. The homeopathic dilution process converts those minerals to energy. The energetic form opens up absorption to help the body develop the structures needed.

The first remedy targets the energy bodies for expansion. The next two remedies are formulas that are given for a week.

The next two remedies are formulas that are given for a week each. During these first 2 weeks, there can be behavioral aggravations, but they usually don't last long and can change daily. One day stubborn, the next day emotional, but they are all related to healing the underlying cause of the problem. Complete change in biochemical function does not come easily.

By the time the child has passed the first two weeks and is taking the remedy that is given for a month, the good changes and gains start to happen. Many kids become functional and able to speak by the end of the 6 weeks. But every one is different. Some only begin to develop pre-speech behaviors such as chewing, blowing, or making noise. Yet many will begin to make gains in cognitive understanding or perception of surroundings. Some will have had no aggravations, while some didn't in the first 2 weeks but do with the month-long remedy. Therefore, I cannot make any general statements about what to expect.

Mostly, the moms are seeing very exciting changes and gains in their children by the end of the six weeks. It seems the greatest gains occur after a particularly difficult aggravation. There can also be changes that occur after the protocol is complete. For this reason, I recommend the parent wait a month before deciding if the remedies worked or not. Some children show no aggravations or gains during the 6 weeks, but begin to improve and develop alertness and speech after finishing the protocol. Older children, 5 to 7 years or more, will take longer to develop fully after the end of the protocol. This is because they are further away from the time the first symptoms appeared. The development of those missing energy structures takes longer than in younger kids.

The world was created in order that the
Perfect Man—the soul of the world—might be
evolved. It is in selfless and humble service to
mankind that man discovers his highest potential.

—Jalal-un-din Rumi, Persian Poet, born 1197.

There is Hope

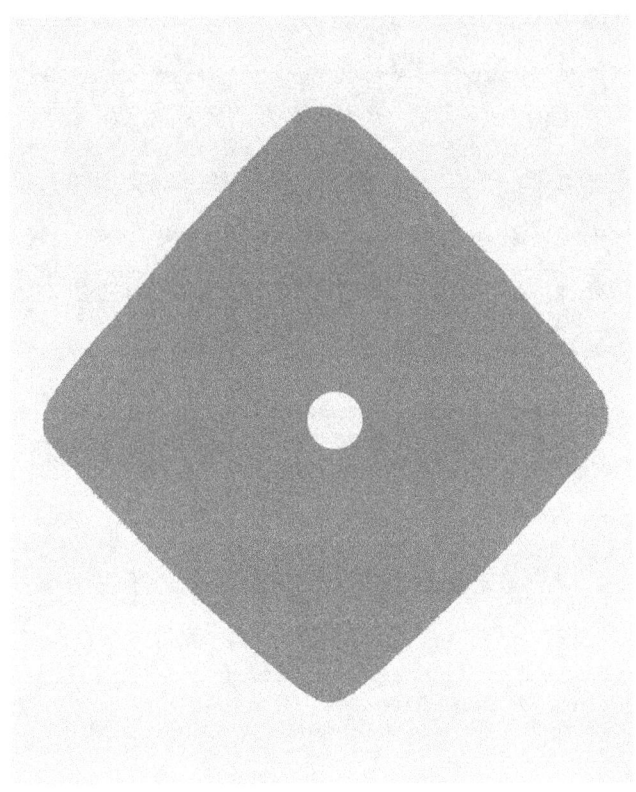

Thoth-ology 201

" I had a very, very dramatic experience with my son when he was 9 months old. He started throwing up, could not keep any food down and turned to skin & bone... ... At the hospital they did every test to him, and in the end just handed him back to me. My wife and I were in bits. The kid was dying...within two weeks (of Homeopathic medicine) he was putting weight on, keeping food down".(The Times, 2008).

— Roger Daltrey

(Lead singer for The Who)

Chapter 17
Classical Homeopathy

If you have tried the remedy program described earlier and are satisfied by the results, you might want to continue to use the healing effects of remedies. You can take control of your life and take care of yourself by learning about the classical system of homeopathy.

Please do not attempt to use homeopathy in serious situations where clearly a medical professional is called for. Homeopathy is for keeping your body in good working order by reversing annoying little problems that many don't consider addressing. In this way, more serious issues can be prevented. These problems may include: allergies, hormonal issues, recurring infections, headaches, digestive issues, stomach pain, minor injury, emotional upheaval and grief.

Do not use homeopathy exclusively and skip doctor visits. To do so is dangerous.

Homeopathy works well in conjunction with conventional treatment and medicines. If your doctor finds a problem, take the medicine prescribed. You can use a remedy to help the body heal the underlying problem afterwards. This strategy can be beneficial in many cases.

The Classical Homeopathic System-Constitution

The original and most often used dosing style in homeopathy is what is commonly called "Classical Homeopathy." The purpose of this system is to find the right constitutional remedy of each individual.

Your constitution is determined to be the state of your entire being, from head to toe, as you were born into this world.

This is also called the "holistic" approach to treatment because it takes a look at the entire person as a whole being, not just a particular area of the body where a problem may be occurring.

A Homeopathic practitioner will find your constitution by looking at signs and symptoms that cover every area of your body. The practitioner will examine the state of your mind, the pains in your head, the condition of your throat, the problems in your stomach, bowels, reproductive organs, and finally your extremities.

All the symptoms over your entire body are analyzed. This analysis is matched to known symptoms of a homeopathic remedy obtained through provings and listed in a Materia Medica. When a match is found, you take that constitutional remedy in a 30th potency for a period of three days only. You do not stop, start over, or repeat that remedy for any reason. The 30th potency remedy starts an energy impulse that travels throughout all parts of you aura and changes the underlying cause of the problem. To stop before the three days is complete, start over or repeat even a single dose of the remedy, would halt the process.

During the three-day-dosing period, you can expect some of your symptoms to aggravate and increase in intensity as your body works them out of your energy bodies. When all aggravations subside, you should experience a new state of health never before realized.

We all come into life with a set of symptoms in a constitutional pattern that deepens as we age, but never really changes until the right constitutional remedy is found and administered.

These patterns are due to many factors that include genetics, learned patterns from family and extended social networks, emotions adopted through experiences, and what we bring with us from past lives.

Our constitutional remedy is the first remedy of choice for any individual. Even unknown problems will shift after that first all-important-dose.

Earlier, I gave an analogy of an orchestra. Your constitution can be likened to the entire orchestra playing a symphony. If individual musicians are not in harmony or playing the wrong music or out of time with the rest of the orchestra, the music will be discordant.

The classically chosen remedy given in a single dose puts everything right again. The system used to find your constitutional remedy can be learned by following the guidelines outlined here and by practice.

Remember, you cannot be harmed by taking the wrong remedy. The worst thing that can happen is that nothing will happen and you are back to where you started.

Aggravations of existing symptoms can, and do, occur. They are a sign that the correct remedy is working on the constitutional problem. Aggravations should last less than 24 hours and leave you with feelings of well-being.

If pain or symptoms lasts for more than 24 hours, it is not an aggravation and has nothing to do with the remedy, but rather a new problem for which the individual must seek medical attention.

Constitutional Dosing

The single-homeopathic-remedy system originating with Samuel Hahnemann and practiced by the prominent American homeopathic doctors of the early 20th Century, is called the Classical System of Homeopathy.

'Single remedy' means that only one remedy is used at a time, in the appropriate potency for the problem, according to the signs and symptoms present in the whole body.

If the problem is not completely cleared, a second remedy must be chosen. The practitioner will reexamine the case and give full consideration to remedies listed as complements—

remedies that have been determined to follow and augment the action of the first remedy—while avoiding those listed as antidotes or remedies that have been found to be detrimental to the action of the original remedy.

Following this system can bring about lasting changes toward normal body function and balance.

A practitioner does not have to memorize millions of symptoms for hundreds of remedies. I certainly have not learned all the symptoms of every one. I find that my mentor's admonition, "Never be so sure of yourself that you think you don't have to look up the symptoms. Never be biased toward a few remedies. Always check the books." is still the "golden rule" of practice.

Learn the Method

Any individual can learn how to use Classical Homeopathy. By using this system in conjunction with the standard homeopathic guides written by James T. Kent and William Boericke, any remedy can be found for any constitutional condition. The use of these guide-books is not as complicated as it would seem by their size and appearance.

The Proper Approach

A medical or allopathic-based approach to using homeopathy attempts to apply allopathic-medical principles in which emphasis is placed on identifying and treating disease instead of focusing on treating symptoms.

It is important to remember that the strength of classical homeopathy lies in its ability to treat all aspects of a person. Homeopathy does not, and never will, work as a treatment for "disease."

Homeopathy is a way to be restored to health and balance through remedies. With homeopathy, it is you who must be treated—not the disease.

With the single remedy system, any symptom, no matter how strange, has a remedy for treatment and becomes a sign to your overall constitution.

Learning to diagnose, understanding the mechanics of disease, or understanding medicine is not required to use common homeopathic remedies. Just follow the rules, matching symptoms to remedies (forget the names of diseases) and you will find that it is possible to relieve nearly any problem.

How to Use The Materia Medica

Many people studying or currently using homeopathic systems are employing computer programs to help in choosing remedies. What follows here is the old- fashioned method of using books. I believe it is beneficial to understand how the books are referenced and the kind of information they contain in order to fully understand the potential of the classical system.

As stated earlier, a homeopathic *Materia Medica* is a book that contains a list of homeopathic remedies and the symptoms they treat.

These symptoms were first caused in provings. A proving is

a kind of test where healthy people take a remedy over a period of time until the symptoms caused by the remedy appear. The symptoms are then recorded.

Homeopathic remedies are chosen for the symptoms they would cause, which is the "like cures like" principle. Due to the "like cures like" principle, homeopathic remedies are known to do the exact opposite of what they would do in a chemical form. For example, coffee is a stimulant, but coffee is a calming remedy when used as Coffea Cruda in the homeopathic form.

William Boericke wrote and published his *Materia Medica* in 1927. He was one of the most prominent homeopathic doctors at the time, and a professor of Homeopathy at the University of California.

Boericke compiled provings from many sources and other *Materia Medica* books of his time to create a handbook that even today is the most useful *Materia Medica* for common use. Look for *Homeopathic Materia Medica* by William Boericke, B. Jain Publishers, India, ISBN 81-7021-003-8. Upon opening the book, you will find the names of the remedies in bold letters and written in Latin. The use of the Latin name for the substance distinguishes the homeopathic remedy from other chemical-based forms of the same substance. The English name is underneath the Latin name in parenthesis.

The first paragraph of each entry contains a general overview of the remedy and the area of the body it works on most prominently. Many also contain information on areas that Boericke had experienced firsthand.

After this first paragraph, there is a list of symptoms arranged in categories according to the areas of the body.

The higher parts of the body come first because they are the most important guiding symptoms. As you look at an entry in the pages, notice the list of symptoms under the 'MIND'. If there is no 'Mind' entry, the list will begin with 'HEAD'.

Most common homeopathic *Materia Medica* books will begin this way. The reason for this is that a remedy will begin its action on the higher parts of the body and move down to lower parts.

Problems in the legs and feet will be listed last because they will be the last symptoms to be relieved when a remedy is taken.

If a problem is purely physical, which means it most likely stems from injury, choose a remedy that describes the physical symptoms best.

If the problem is biochemical—allergies, arthritis, sleep, etc.—be sure to match the mental symptoms under the 'MIND' heading to the person being treated.

This doesn't necessarily mean that mental symptoms will change unless that is the problem being treated, but in many cases, the mental makeup is the major guide to the correct remedy.

There is a small repertory in the back of *Boericke's Materia Medica*. In the Indian Publication (the B. Jain publication printed in India) it begins on page 689.

A repertory is a list of symptoms, followed by a list of remedies that have those symptoms in its proving.

The symptom categories in the repertory also start with the mind, followed by the head, and on down the body to the extremities.

On the first page of the repertory (p. 689), the first symptom listed is AWKWARD-Lets things fall from hand. Remedies are listed after that in alphabetical order, and abbreviated. Since the Materia Medica is also in alphabetical order, it is not difficult to find the remedies, even if you do not understand the abbreviation.

In Boericke's Repertory, the remedies in italics are more important and have a stronger affinity to the symptoms than remedies in regular type.

In the listing for AWKWARD—**Apis, Bov**, and *Nat.M* are in italics. If you wanted to find the remedy that most matched your awkward person, you would go to each of these remedies in the *Materia Medica* until you were satisfied with one remedy that matched most of characteristics of the person.

Go to the *Materia Medica* section of the book and turn to 'Apis' on page 61. The first sentence in that entry tells you where the remedy has the most influence. Read through the symptoms.

Don't be inhibited by medical terminology. Most entries are common sense and easy to read. The entries in italics are more important than those in regular type. If you can find five to six sentences throughout the list of symptoms that match the symptoms of the person who is in need of treatment, it is well-indicated. The person doesn't have to display all the symptoms in each category, just one, and five to six other symptoms from the overall entry for a particular remedy.

For example, if a person matches the:

"awkward; drops things readily" symptom in the 'MIND'

"vertigo worse when closing the eyes" in the 'HEAD'

"stinging pains" in the 'THROAT'

"extremely tender" symptoms in the 'ABDOMEN'

and "hoarseness" in the 'RESPIRATORY', it would be a well-indicated remedy and should relieve not only these problems but many more which were not necessarily thought of as problems. If you can find other symptoms that match, the remedy is even more indicated.

Practice

The more you practice looking up symptoms in the repertory and reading remedies in the *Materia Medica*, the more familiar you become with remedies and matching them to symptoms.

Start with any symptom in any part of the body, but it should be the most prominent physical symptom—the one giving the most pain or the biggest problem.

It seems to work best to choose a physical symptom to look up first rather than a mental one because physical symptoms are typically more distinctive.

Next, find the symptom in the repertory. Look at the list of remedies and find those that are italicized. Then turn to the *Materia Medica* section of the book and study each remedy, until you find the one that matches the most symptoms over all.

You can't miss finding the remedy that will be most helpful when you use this method.

Be sure to match a mental symptom in the Mind section to the person being studied. It may not be what you start with when you look up symptoms in the repertory, but it is still the most important guiding symptom. Your rate of success will be much higher if you do this.

Kent's Repertory—*The Repertory of the*
Homeopathic Materia Medica

(B. Jain Publishers of India, ISBN 81-7021-059-3) written by Dr. James T. Kent can be used in the same way to complement the *Materia Medica*. Kent's Repertory is a huge work, covering a great many symptoms. If you are interested in homeopathy and wish to continue to study, I recommend Kent's book.

To use the repertory, look up the symptoms one by one, starting with the higher parts of the body and moving to lower areas. In other words, the symptom of a headache is more important than the symptom of foot pain, unless the foot pain in the most prominent symptom.

As you find a particular symptom with a characteristic quality, such as a 'pain in the forehead that throbs' you will see a list of all the remedies that describe that type of pain.

As you read further in the column, you will see more and more specific situations where that pain may occur. This gives you possible and idiosyncratic symptoms in order to match the best situation to the person suffering the pain.

The remedies written in bold print are the most often used remedies for that symptom, italicized remedies are the next most common, and the remedies written in plain print are the least often used. However, if you find a specific situation, such as 'pain in the forehead that throbs when lying in the dark' and there is only one remedy listed, and that remedy is written in plain print, it will still be a perfect match to the person's constitution. Consulting the *Materia Medica* will confirm that there are symptoms related to that person in multiple headings of that specific remedy.

New Symptoms

After the remedy you have chosen is taken, the symptoms may be relieved, but it is also possible for a new symptom to become prominent.

When this happens, more than one remedy is required for complete relief. Look up the new symptoms in the repertory. Read the remedies listed under it, and find a match to the new problems, again matching the mental symptom as well.

Relationships

In the back of *Boericke's Materia Medica* starting on page 1080 (of the B. Jain publication) there is a chart called **"The Relationship of Remedies with Duration of Action."**

Find the remedy you took first in the left hand column. Next, look to see if there is a relationship to the remedy you plan to take next.

If the new remedy is found in the column labeled "Complements" or "Remedies that Follow Well," you can expect good results because the second remedy helps to continue and promote the reaction begun by the first.

"Inimicals" are remedies that do not follow each other well and will give an adverse reaction. Be certain that you do **not** use an inimical after your first remedy.

Antidotes can also be compatibles, but taking an antidote to the first remedy will stop any further beneficial action.

If two remedies have no relationship, there is no problem in taking one after the other.

Be Patient

The column that has the **"Duration"** of the remedy's action is important. Each remedy has a duration of action. That means that if you take one dose or several, the reaction will continue in your body for the number of days listed in the column.

This does not mean you take it for the number of days listed. It means that you must consider when taking a remedy that it will continue working for only one day or sixty days depending on its nature.

Anything you take after the first remedy should be compatible with it. If it is not, the curative action may be interrupted. It also means that you should be patient and let the remedies work.

Many times the strongest action takes place up to a week after you have completed a remedy. It may be difficult, but resist the temptation to take more and more remedies. That is the way conventional medicine works and this is not conventional medicine.

With homeopathy, the effect is just the opposite. You take a little and the action can continue for a long time afterwards. The problem doesn't return when you stop taking the remedy as it can with herbs or conventional medicine.

How to Take Remedies

In general:

- 6th potency is taken three times a day for a month

- 12th potency is taken three times a day for a week.

- 30th potency is taken three times a day for three days.

- 200th potency is taken in one dose only.
  Or multiple times in acute dosing.

- 1M or 1000 potency is taken in one dose only.

- A constitutional remedy is taken in a 30th
  potency for three days only and not repeated.

After the doses are taken, let them act. You will notice symptoms come and go then subside completely as the remedy works its curative action.

If an uncomfortable aggravation occurs, take an extra dose to help the body work through the problem. This is particularly effective for formulas or 6th potency single remedies. This is more effective than stopping the remedy as you would with an allopathic treatment. Remember, there is no drug side effect with homeopathy, just an energy impulse clearing the problem.

To take a homeopathic remedy, place 2 or 3 of the pellets under the tongue and let them dissolve.

Do not have anything in your mouth fifteen minutes before

and after taking the remedy. Do not swallow the pellets down the throat as you do with pills—just place them dry under the tongue and let them dissolve. It is okay if small children chew them. Dissolve them in an ounce of water for small babies who can't yet chew.

Caution in Repeating Remedies

If your symptoms have gone away but return in a changed form, you may repeat the same remedy taken earlier, but with caution. If you repeat the same remedy while its duration of action is still working, you can antidote the effect and it will be difficult to get a good reaction started again. It would be better to take a complement remedy before repeating, so the actions of the two doses of the same remedy don't clash. Another more preferable course is to move to the next higher potency of the same remedy.

For example, if you took Arsenicum Album 30C for an allergy, and it went away for a while, but returned within a short period of time but in a lesser or slightly different form, do not repeat Arsenicum 30C right away. The action of Arsenicum can continue acting for 60 to 90 days. The actual duration varies from one individual to the next.

The first dose can bring up multiple minor aggravations while it is working on old problems embedded in your energy bodies. Repeating the same potency while the first dose is still acting will cause the energy of those doses to smash into each other, ending the action of both and making it difficult to get that remedy to work for you again.

As an example, if you found that you needed to repeat Arsenicum, it would be better to take a complement such as Apis or Belladonna to offset the action of the first dose.

If the symptoms you took Arsenicum for never return, do not repeat it for at least several months—and only if new symptoms lead you to choose it for a different problem.

Once a remedy has worked, repeating it while it is still active will bring back the problems—perhaps permanently. So, if you are tempted to help a remedy along since it did so well to help the first time—don't.

The Potency is Too High

Continuing with the example of Arsenicum, if a 30th potency worked for a short period of time but symptoms returned exactly as they were in the beginning, it may be that the 30th was too high to get to the affected energy body. You cannot take a lower potency of the same remedy straight away, since taking the lower potency of the same remedy would cause the remedy to collapse and drain, according to the effects of a chord potency (see Chords in Chapter 18). You could use a complement first, then drop to a lower potency of Arsenicum such as a 12th and see if that helps relieve the symptoms on a more permanent basis.

Since Arsenicum Album is a poison in its unpotentized state, it is not commonly available nor is it advisable to take it in a potency lower than a 9X or 6C.

Antidotes

You may have read or been told by others who use homeopathy that strong smelling substances will antidote remedies. Many people avoid trying homeopathy because the restrictions and the diet they think must be followed while under homeopathic care. These restrictions often seem overly austere. In fact, homeopathic remedies are energetic and are not impacted by substances in the physical realm. Even the 6th potency is energetically high enough to not be affected by material substances.

There is a chart on Page 1080 of the B. Jain publication of *Boericke's Materia Medica* (The Gibson Miller Chart) that gives the duration of action for each remedy, along with a list of antidotes.

Some remedies, for example, list COFF. as an antidote. Where this is listed, the remedy could be antidoted by COFFEA CRUDA as a homeopathic remedy, but not by coffee as the gross material substance you drink in the morning.

Homeopathics and Environmental Factors

Homeopathic remedies should not be exposed to excessive heat (temperatures over 150 degrees F.), cold (below freezing), nor contaminated by food items (such as juice being spilled on them). Nor should they be placed in containers that have been previously used for another purpose. Beyond these cautions, there is nothing that will affect the action of a homeopathic remedy. After it is taken, what you eat or drink does not matter as long as it is not within fifteen minutes before or after taking the remedy.

When a remedy is working, nothing material will antidote it. I have never known a well chosen remedy to be easily antidoted by normal life activities.

Caffeine, for instance, is not a problem as some people have been led to believe, nor is mint toothpaste if it is not used within fifteen minutes of taking the remedy.

Blame

Some homeopathic practitioners have blamed common substances for antidoting remedies as a way to explain why a remedy didn't work. These homeopathic practitioners are likely in the habit of using high potencies for physical problems. If the potency is too high, it skirts by the energy body affected, giving a temporary amelioration of symptoms, but symptoms will return if the potency was too high—not because it was antidoted by a material substance.

On the Web

It is actually quite easy to find the homeopathic books, Amazon carries many. Amazon also carries many of the common remedies. One of my favorite websites to order Boiron remedies from is www.healthland.com

More Information

If you wish to do more research, there are a multitude of web sites dedicated to homeopathy and the experiences of individuals using remedies.

Be cautious, although there is much information about alternative and complementary health on the Internet, much of it does not reflect reliable research nor is it the voice of experienced practitioners but rather a sounding board for personal opinions, theories, and hidden agendas.

Before making any decisions about trying an alternative health care system, research thoroughly and consult with highly rated, reputable professionals.

In 1987 Cher was struck by a debilitating viral illness that manifested in chronic fatigue and pneumonia. "I tried regular medicine and it just didn't work...I turned to a Homeopathic doctor in desperation... within four months he'd got me back up and on the road again". (Sloan, 2004).

—Cher (Singer, Entertainer, Actress)

Chapter 18

Combinations VS. Single Remedies

Through the years, various homeopathy professionals have attempted to simplify the process of choosing the right remedy and potency for each individual. Many have designed memory schemes to allow a practitioner to know which remedies to recommend for each problem. Others have attempted to discover a "magic" formula to calculate the strength of each potency so the exact strength needed can be determined. Most of these researchers and reformers have recognized the impossibility of holding in memory, the massive amount of information to make proper remedy and potency choices for each client. Therefore, many have streamlined the process by creating combinations.

Some combinations were created by combining multiple remedies into a single preparation. If, for example, there are five remedies helpful for migraine headaches, all five are combined into a single product and sold for migraine headaches.

You can buy these combinations anytime without the advice or help from a practitioner. There are many useful combinations on the market for specific, short-term acute illness and symptoms. These can help you feel better by quickly alleviating symptoms—often bringing relief not possible from over-the-counter, chemically-based medications.

Combination remedies can be a good choice for immediate relief of simple problems. In cases where a homeopathic practitioner is not readily available, these combinations allow you to select a homeopathic preparation based on a simple understanding of the package instructions. These preparations can allow you to discover some of the many benefits possible with homeopathic treatments.

Their safety makes these remedies, in most cases, preferable over chemically-based, over-the-counter products which can have unintended side effects.

Not For Long Term Use

Combinations are not meant for long-term use or chronic problems. They will not change biochemistry to bring about lasting relief from chronic problems. The reason for this limitation lies in the way the remedies are combined and how they interact with each other.

Homeopathic Chords

Some combinations are multiple potencies of the same remedy— known as chords. These preparations contain a single remedy. However, instead of a single potency, the preparation may contain multiple potencies that have been placed into the same pellet. A typical chord may contain potencies of 3C, 12C, 30C, and 60C.

At the time these chord remedies were developed, it was believed the potencies would remain separate and not blend into one large potency, or perhaps average themselves out to a mid-range level. Many homeopaths who lacked a full understanding of how to select potencies, believed that combinations could simplify the process of choosing because a body would select the right one and the others would simply vanish.

According to one theory, if it is difficult to choose a correct potency, many in one remedy can provide the correct one, and the vibration level of each individual patient would take only the one needed. That is not what happens.

Another theory touts ease of administration. It is unnecessary to change potency during the course treatment. The resonating potency will correctly match the problem because it changes vibration levels during its course of action.

Another theory is that your body can average the chords to create a potency not found in the original combination. For example, in a Calcarea Carb. chord your body could average the 3C and the 12C to create a 7C. It was also believed that your body could create any potency needed simply by adding together the full range in the chord. In the example of Calcarea Carb. your body would be able to create any potency from 3C to 105C based on its ability to add them together.

Unfortunately, all of these theories were based on a chemical model that is not applicable in homeopathy.

Chords were first described in the early twentieth century by Dr. Cadiz, of Barcelona, Spain. He prepared and used single remedies in multiple potencies. He likened them to musical chords, and discovered that the therapeutic action of the multiple potencies worked differently from single ones. It wasn't until the 1970s that the application of these remedies became widespread and a variety of theories concerning their use became apparent.

Not the Way it Seems

Energy has its own properties and does not obey chemical laws. In chemistry, all compounds added together have a cumulative and interacting effect. However, each energy signature remains distinct and unique. The energy of potentized remedies does not blend together to create a cumulative effect. Because of the unique property of energy, the combination of potencies is acting in a unique way.

When lower potencies are combined with higher potencies in a combination chord, the lower ones fall through the platform created by the higher, because the lower potencies are heavier. All but the lowest potencies drain out of your body. Not only are none of the higher potencies left to work, the falling through effect will actually drain away a previously helpful single remedy.

Any curative effect from a chord will be found in its lowest potency, which will remain after all higher ones have drained.

There are times when the drainage effect from a multiple potency is desirable, such as with Zinc or lead, but it is important to know what is really happening.

For example, a multiple potency chord of Zincum Metalicum could be helpful in draining an excess accumulations of zinc, which can cause pain in the heels of the feet, but chords are not appropriate when a remedy needs to remain in the body.

When Not to Use a Chord

A friend of mine once suffered a severe head trauma from a car accident. This caused seizures. For years she used calcium antacids in an attempt to control the seizures. As a result, she suffered constant stomach acidity.

I suggested Calcarea Carb. as a homeopathic form of calcium—instead of antacids. Calcarea Carb. would be more readily absorbed by her cells that needed the calcium.

After her first course of treatment with Calcarea Carb. in a 30th potency, three times a day for three days, she reported that the acidity in her stomach had gone and she stopped taking the antacids. She was also completely free of seizures.

This lasted for several months until she tried a product being marketed by a new company—a remedy of Calcarea Carb. in a chord potency with 3C, 12C, 30C, 60C all together. The beneficial effects she had received from homeopathic calcium was wiped out by this product. The stomach acidity and seizures returned. The calcium that had been put in place by the single remedy was drained by the chord.

The Drainage Effect

Homeopathic potencies, when given one at a time, arrange themselves on top of each other, similar to a stack of layers on a cake. Because the lower potencies are heavier (they contain more of the original substance) they move into place at a slower speed and must be allowed to settle into place before the next lighter (higher) faster potency is added.

In multiple potency combinations, the top layers move into place faster than the heavier lower layers. This arrangement is much like placing the smaller layers onto the cake plate before adding the larger layers, which results in an unstable structure that will collapse the entire cake. To keep potencies in the body, they must be built up from lower to higher attenuations, just as a cake—the lighter layers on top of the heavier ones.

Lower potencies collapse through lighter, higher potencies and drain out. Using lower potencies first and building to higher creates a stable foundation.

This means that if multiple potencies are required for a particular problem, the remedies must be given in a lower 6th first. A 30th of the same remedy may follow, and a 200th can be given after that. I sometimes use this method with Stramonium to expand the energy bodies in individuals who have internalized their energy structures. Stramonium in 30th potency first, followed a few days later with a single dose of the 200th potency, followed later with a single dose of the 1M potency, and then the 10M potency a few days after, allow energy bodies and levels to expand.

If you start with a higher potency, say a 30th, then step down to a lower, such as a 6th straight away, the effect will be drainage.

Substance Overload

There are times when a problem is caused by an overload of a certain substance. Even a needed nutrient can create overload if consumed in excess or over a prolonged period of time.

In a case of overload, a chord of the offending substance will help drain it from your body. The lowest potency that remains helps resolve problems with absorption or detoxification— depending on whether the substance is essential or harmful.

Some combinations are multiple remedies in multiple potencies. These are used for draining toxic substances. Like any other combination, there is a time and a place where they are useful. These combinations are best for draining toxins such as petroleum, phenol chemicals, heavy metals, and other pollutants, but they will not bring about permanent changes in biochemistry unless the undesirable state was caused by your reaction to the original pollutant.

In these cases, draining the toxins allows your body to return to its original state of balanced normality. However, if the original physical state—before the toxin was introduced— was unbalanced, removing the toxin will not correct the original problem.

If your body is functioning properly, elimination will take place automatically. Our physical bodies have amazing abilities to detox without help if allowed to do so. Unless the condition is incurable, single remedies can bring you back into proper function.

What is Health?

It can be a dangerous mistake to believe we are intrinsically sick and have to be colon-cleansed, de-parasited, de-toxed, and over-vitamined to be healthy.

While these popular therapies may be called for when we truly have a dysfunction or illness, their overuse by symptom-free individuals can be harmful.

You simply have to allow your body to carry out its natural functions in the way it was designed to do—gently and easily.

A well-chosen, single remedy, given in the correct potency, will create a solid, stable, lasting effect.

Single Remedies

A single remedy taken alone, without any other remedy mixed with it or combined with other single remedies is best. Other single remedies can be taken close to the same time, but not in the same dose.

If you desire to take more than one single remedy in a short period of time, take the remedy, wait 15 minutes for it to absorb then eat something or drink a sip of water to close down the portal under the tongue. Wait another 15-minutes before taking the next remedy. In this way, the two single remedies will not mix, and the beneficial effect of the two will be achieved.

Impatience

Often, seeking instantaneous results, a client will insist upon a second dose or an additional remedy before allowing sufficient time for the first one to fully manifest.

Sometimes, a practitioner, perhaps new to the field of homeopathy or desperately wishing to help a client in distress, will be tempted to prescribe multiple remedies simultaneously or over a short period of time. Another mistake is to prescribe a remedy to be taken periodically, say once a week. This method will most often antidote the effect of the remedy.

A remedy should not be repeated during its duration of action. The remedy determines how long it will act—not the potency. Only 6X potencies or combination formulas are unaffected by duration.

Even if symptoms return or increase during the duration of action, the remedy may still be present and acting. It is important to remember that a well-chosen remedy can often produce an aggravation (an increase in symptoms) as it pushes the problem or condition out of the physical body and energy bodies.

If Symptoms Return

In a case where the problem is only partially cleared or it is gone and returns after a short period of time, it is probably because the potency was wrong.

Symptoms return because the potency is incorrect and working on the wrong energy level—not because the remedy has stopped working or was interrupted by a material substance.

Different potencies will work on different energy levels, but it is the remedy that will work over a period of time. For some remedies it is one day. Others work for a week or two. Most of the multi-symptom, deep acting constitutional remedies work for 30 to 60, even 90 days.

Even if symptoms return, a remedy should not be repeated during this duration, nor should the practitioner hurry to select an additional remedy unless new symptoms indicate the use of a different one.

R. Gibson Miller compiled a chart that gives duration of action information. This chart is located in the back of the publications from India (B. Jain Publishers LTD of India) of *Boericke's Materia Medica* **(pages 1079 to 1097), and** *Kent's Repertory of the Materia Medica* **(pages 1437 to 1455).**

Lower Potency

No matter what the potency, do not repeat the same remedy in a lower potency. The energy of the lower one will fall through the higher and cause both to drain out of the body. This can be true for the entire duration of the remedy. If you wish to repeat a remedy within its duration, go to the next higher potency, never lower.

For example, if you have a calcium absorption issue, use 30th potency. If you want to switch to the 6X of the **same** remedy, it is important to remember to use other remedies in between the two potencies of the same substance.

If another remedy is used in between the two potencies of the same remedy, the rule for never going to a lower potency in the same remedy does not apply. Lycopodium Clavitum is often a good remedy choice for this purpose.

If your symptoms go away for a while, but come back in a short time, the potency was probably too high. It went to an energy and level above the problem, giving you only temporary relief. This can be likened to mowing a lawn to get rid of dandelions. It may remove all of the yellow flowers, but they will simply return because the roots are still present.

Remedy compliments are listed in the back of *Boericke's Materia Medica* and Kent's Repertory, in the Miller chart, but only in the version from India printed by B. Jain Publications. The books published by Boericke and Tafel in Santa Rosa, California do not carry this information.

Remedy Antidotes

A list of remedy antidotes is also in the Miller chart. These refer to potentized antidotes. Chemical-based substances will not antidote a homeopathically potentized remedy because they do not act on the same energy level.

If a remedy has stopped working, it has not come in contact with an antidote. It has been given in the wrong potency. Since traditional homeopaths have not addressed potency interaction on energy bodies, it seemed reasonable for them to blame outside interference by certain substances as the reason why remedies stopped working.

Taboos about using coffee, caffeine, chocolate, camphor, eucalyptus, mint, and a variety of other strong smelling substances while using a homeopathic remedy are common. If all those prohibitions were actually factors in antidoting remedies, few would have benefited from homeopathy during its long history. Chemicals and odors do not antidote potentized remedies. Remedies stop working due to incorrect use of potency.

Chapter 19

Zinc Drainage

Recent research suggests that some people who suffer from anorexia are low in zinc. This initial problem may be the result of an inability to absorb dietary zinc or to process it into a usable form.

Adding zinc to diet cannot correct this malfunction. No matter how much is added, if you cannot absorb and process it, the deficiency and the resulting anorexia will continue. Zinc deficiency suppresses appetite. Correcting this deficiency and absorption issue homeopathically can eliminate anorexic behavior.

Early in my homeopathic practice, I saw a client with an anorexia-type problem. She complained that she wasn't able to eat because food had become repulsive. She had no appetite and was fearful that her battle with food was serious. I suggested she try a dose of homeopathically potentized zinc—Zincum Metalicum.

She took a 6X potency for a week. A month or so later she came to see me again for a different problem. She reported that her anorexia had completely disappeared. Her appetite returned and she had gained a few pounds.

Zinc and Overeating

In the same way an imbalance caused by an inability to absorb zinc can create anorexia, an inability to eliminate zinc can manifest as a weight related problem. Deficiency is related to anorexia or food avoidance. Zinc overload can bring on compulsive over eating.

In 1995 a patent was issued for an antimicrobial zinc lozenge and marketed as a cure for common cold symptoms. Perhaps ironically, the first zinc lozenge product on the market used homeopathically potentized zinc. That particular product boosted the immune system without causing zinc accumulation.

Many people who used the zinc lozenges in non-homeopathic material dosages found their lymphatic systems clogged, a reduced immune response and weight gain. This is all due to zinc accumulation in the body.

Additional sources for excess zinc can stem from the belief that all supplements must contain balanced nutrients at levels often far exceeding the recommended daily allowance. The overwhelming belief that everyone must take daily supplements in order to avoid vitamin deficiencies contributes to the zinc overload.

Diet is not the only source of zinc. Zinc oxide is often used as a preventative and treatment for diaper rash, eczema, psoriasis, sunburn and other skin aliments. Many forms of zinc are commonly found in products such as sun blocks, make-up, and as an all-natural coloring agent in consumables, all of which contribute to zinc overload. The presence of zinc in personal care products is not a bad thing, since zinc is a necessary nutrient. But, it becomes a problem when we can't eliminate excess zinc.

As zinc accumulates, it becomes toxic. If you cannot eliminate the excess, your body compensates by increasing appetite and lowering your metabolism.

Why some bodies forget how to properly process and eliminate zinc is related to calcium absorption deficiency. The two problems go hand in hand, but why is not yet clear.

Weight Problems and Excess Zinc

As zinc accumulates, it becomes toxic. If you cannot eliminate the excess, your body compensates by increasing appetite and lowering your metabolism. This causes you to gain weight. This is your body's attempt to dilute excess zinc with an increase in body mass.

Unfortunately, as you eat more or take more supplements, you consume more zinc. If you diet, you increase the concentration of it in your system since zinc is then liberated from the fat. This will cause you to crave food to dilute the zinc with body bulk. It's a never-ending cycle.

This syndrome is so common it has its own name—Yo-Yo dieting. It is a major problem, yet the allopathic medical community has no adequate means to address it.

The homeopathic system, on the other hand, has several techniques that address the original malfunction. One technique is to get rid of the excess zinc overload.

Draining the Zinc

The concept of Cord remedies discussed earlier is critical in addressing issues such as zinc deficiency and overload. By using the correct potencies of precise remedies, in individually designed programs, it is possible to correct the underlying cause of weight gain. By taking the proper remedies, you will not only drain excess zinc out of your body, but also correct any mal-absorption problem. When this occurs, your cells will absorb zinc as a nutrient, stop the excess storage, and allow you to begin to get rid of excess weight.

Eliminating Toxins

In some people, homeopathic remedies have an immediate impact on weight reduction—often beginning with the very first remedies. More often, however, the remedies make changes in mineral absorption and shift in biochemistry that enable other weight control programs to work more effectively. This allows you to obtain and maintain optimum weight levels without suffering the Yo-Yo syndrome.

Success Stories

The problem with conventional weight loss programs is that they release toxins stored in your fat cells. This can overload your body with toxins and other substances causing override mechanisms to kick in to neutralize excess levels. Your appetite increases and you regain .

Homeopathic remedies for weight control have subtle but definite effects. For example, I had a case where the client, by balancing zinc, had a steady decrease in appetite, loss of the fear of hunger, the ability to be "choosy" about food rather than simply consuming anything presented—as well as the ability to leave food on the plate after reaching a point of satisfaction. This client remarked that for the first time food was a choice and not a need.

In another case, also after balancing zinc, the client's intense need for food, that had been unrelated to hunger, had diminished.

He also reported that he'd lost his fear of physical activity and started to enjoy being active.

Another client reported that she couldn't remember a time in her life that she didn't dread the idea of exercising. After balancing her zinc, she enjoyed the feeling of moving her body.

A woman I saw a few years ago for zinc overload, had the expected decrease in appetite, and a new feeling of mental clarity. She told me that she'd been asked by a therapist, "What do you think about while you're eating?" Food and anger were so linked in her that it was impossible to eat without getting angry. She also couldn't get angry without eating.

After taking the appropriate remedy, that connection between anger and food was broken. She said that for the first time that she could remember, she could eat and simply enjoy the experience. She also reported that when she became upset or angry she no longer found herself eating compulsively.

Mental Changes

Mental changes associated with the homeopathic treatment of zinc accumulation occur because higher level potencies of homeopathic remedies act in the upper energy levels. In the case of zinc drainage, the 30th potency is acting on higher energy levels to drain excess zinc from brain tissue where it can accumulate as a pollutant and clog mental function and cause cloudy thinking.

Draining excess zinc from the mental realms often results in your body using zinc correctly for mental function. The sensation of fog lifting from the mind brings new understanding of old thinking patterns.

Caution

If you use homeopathic remedies to help correct a weight control problem, there is a possible side effect related to the decreased consumption of food. As your appetite lessens, the amount of food, water, and other fluids you consume also decreases. Food is a major source of fluid. Be aware that decreasing your intake of food could bring a temporary, slight dehydration.

Compensate by increasing the amount of fluids you consume, particularly at the beginning of a program. Because of the balancing action from homeopathic remedies, the likelihood that this problem will occur is slight. If it does occur, it is normally short-lived and seldom presents any serious problems.

Remember to use normal caution when exercising, participating in strenuous activity, or simply conducting normal activity in hot weather. Remember to compensate with extra fluids for the loss of them from decreased food consumption and to replace those you lose through sweating.

When taking zinc drainage remedies, it is not unusual to experience a temporary soreness and swelling in lymph glands, particularly if you have been taking zinc lozenges or zinc supplements. This is because zinc accumulates in the glands— including salivary and prostate. The drainage remedy system will purge accumulated zinc, causing glandular soreness and swelling.

After the initial purging, you may actually begin to feel proper lymph response when your immune system is fighting off an infection or an invading virus.

Another common sign of zinc accumulation is pain in the heels when stepping or walking. If zinc drainage brings relief, the return of the pain would signal a new accumulation of zinc and a need to repeat the drainage remedies.

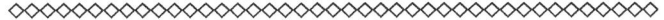

And there you have it, everything I believe to be true about the energetic action of homeopathic remedies and how energy works to improve health and wellbeing—Thoth-ology in theory and practice.

Notes

Title Quote

1. Rupert Sheldrake, 2012, p. 12

Preface

1. Hughes, 1993, p.609

2. Iqbal, 1908, p.30

Chapter 1

1. Sheldrake, 2012, p. 31-32

2. Sheldrake, 2012, p. 33

3. Qureshi, 1980

4. Hahnemann, 1997, p. 97

5. Sheldrake, 2012, p. 49

6. Sheldrake, 2012, p. 99

7. Sheldrake, 2012, p. 100

8. Lipton, 2005, p.61

9. Lipton, 2005, p.61-62

Chapter 2

1. Bruce Lipton (The Biology of Belief, 2005)
   Lynne McTaggart (The Field, 2002)

2. Figure 1.1, Sheldrake, 2012, p. 50

3. Iqbal, 2012

4. Sheldrake, 2012, p. 214

5. Iqbal, 2012

6. Dean Radin (Supernormal, 2013)

7. Lipton, 2005, p.55

8. Lipton, 2005, p.100

9. Iqbal, (1908)

Chapter 3

1. Lipton, 2005, p. 53-54

2. Sheldrake, 2012, p. 99

3. Hahnemann, 1997, p.103

Chapter 4

1. Hahnemann, 1997, Paragraph 272, p. 296

2. O'Reilly, 1996, p.77

Chapter 5

1. Qureshi, (1980)

2. Hahnemann, 1997

References:

Boericke,(1995) William, M.D., Homeopathic Materia Medica and Repertor

B. Jain Publishers, New Delhi,India, Reprint Edition 1995

Carroll, (2010) Lee, Kryon Book Twelve, Platinum Publishing House, P. 102

Clark, (1978) J.H., A Dictionary of Practical Materia Medica by John Henry Clark, M.D., London 1900. Published by B. Jain Publishers, New Delhi, page 178

Freely, (2009) John, Aladdin's Lamp, How Greek Science Came to Europe Through the Islamic World, Random House, New York, P. 58

Handley, Rima, A Homeopathic Love Story, North Atlantic Books, Berkeley, CA1990

Hughes, (1965) Thomas Patrick, A Dictionary of Islam, Reference Book
Publishers, New Jersey 1965, first published in India in 1883, P. 609

Hahnemann,(1997) Samuel, William Boericke's English translation, Organon of
Medicine, BJain Publishers, India.

Iqbal, (1908) Allama Muhammad, The Development of Metaphysics in Persia,
A Contribution to the History of Muslim Philosophy, Luzac and Co. London 1908,reprinted by Sang-E-Meel Publications, Lahore, Pakistan, (2004) PP. 30-52

Iqbal, (2012) Michele, "How to Choose Potency", The Homeopathic Heritage,
Bringing Classical and Contemporary Homeopathy Together, Vol. 38, No. 07, New Delhi, India, October 2012

Kent,(1995) J.T., Repertory of the Homoeopathic Materia Medica, B. Jain Publishers, New Delhi, India, Reprint Edition 1995.

Lipton, (2005) Bruce,The Biology of Belief, Unleashing the Power of
    Consciousness, Matter and Miracles, Hay House, INC.

Lyon, (1978) Albert s. Medicine: An Illustrated History, Henry N. Abrams Inc. New York,

McTaggart, (2002) Lynne, The Field: The Quest for the Secret Force of the
    Universe. P.104 Harper Collins, New York.

Milgram, (2007) Lionel, "Toward a United Theory of Homeopathy and Conventional
    Medicine" The Journal of Alternative and Complementary Medicine, Vol. 13,
    Number 7, pp. 759-769.

O'Reilly, (1996) Wenda Brewster, Organon of the Medical Art by Dr. Samuel
    Hahnemann, Birdcage Books, Redmond, Washington, P.77

Qureshi, (1980) Masood, Principles of Homeopathy for Medical Students, Masood

Publications, Lahore, Pakistan

Radin, (2013) Dean, Supernatural: Science, Yoga, and the Evidence for

Extraordinary Psychic Abilities. Random House, New York.

Sheldrake, (1995) Rupert, A new science of life: The hypothesis of morphic resonance, Rochester, Vermont: Park Street Press.

Sheldrake, (2012) Rupert, Science Set Free: 10 Paths to New Discovery. Random

House, New York.

About the Author

Dr. Iqbal's family background is basically of Irish descent and originally from the State of Washington. She grew up in the Seattle area, but went to high school in Sacramento, CA. She finished college at U.C. Davis, wheres he met her husband, Muhammad.

In 1982, they were living in Pakistan when she met her first homeopathic doctor and began the journey to learn all she could about homeopathy in order to take care of her children. In 1987, she completed a four-year- Ph.D. equivalent program at the National College of Homeopathy in Rawalpindi, a branch of the National Council of Homeopathy of Pakistan. Due to political changes in Pakistan that took place in 1988, Dr. Iqbal and her family decided to come back to the States. They have been living in Southern California since 1989.

Dr. Iqbal had taught ESL while living in Pakistan, and upon returning to California she decided that to become a teacher. It was not to be. In 1995, she left all of her teaching jobs and went to work for Capitol Drugs on Santa Monica Blvd in West Hollywood. Capitol Drugs was one of the first homeopathic pharmacies in Southern California after remedies became available to the public in 1989. She worked at the pharmacy for five years.

After Capitol Drugs, she started a homeopathic practice in the Riverside area of Southern California. Dr. Iqbal continues to practice in Riverside.

www.ingramcontent.com/pod-product-compliance
Lightning Source LLC
Chambersburg PA
CBHW060243290526
45789CB00001B/166